Melanoma without a Cause

*How the New Miracle Immunotherapy
Drugs and My Own Immune System
Helped Me Fight Stage Four Cancer*

BRYANT WIENEKE

TO ELVIRA ROSE, WITH LOVE

Acknowledgements

It's not often you get to thank someone for saving your life, so here goes:

Thank you, Elvira, for being there every step of the way and holding me up for many of those steps. Thank you to Michael, Brian and Rachel; Aurora and Frank; my brother, Steve; Kim, Gilbert and Geronimo; the Crafty Women (Alicia, Lynn, Marie, and Nicole); Sister Fran and the Daughters of Charity; Tina and the Monastery of Poor Clares; Alfred and his men's prayer group; Simran Singh, Amrita and Simran Bindra; Roger and Sheryl; John and Mary; Sergio and Eloy; Matt, Ben and Oliver; and all our other wonderfully supportive family and friends, many of whom are mentioned in the journal. Thank you to Dr. Mark Abate; Dr. Bruce Kendle; the kind and brave RNs and other doctors and staff of the Sansum Clinic Oncology/Hematology Department; Dr. Gayatri Heesen; Karen Hannah Arndt, PA-C; Santa Barbara Sansum Clinic; Cottage Hospital ER staff and Oncology Floor; HealthNet; and Bristol-Myers Squibb. A special shout-out goes to Professor James Allison and the other researchers involved in the development of immunotherapy drugs. You are heroes. And while perhaps not heroic, Ann Sonstelie's editing is much appreciated, and so is the input from Alan, Ginna, James, and Roxanne.

PART ONE: A NEW REALITY

THE CALL NOBODY WANTS

When I was eight years old, I began to have waves of terror break over me at bedtime. I was not scared of monsters in the closet or boogie men peeking through the windows. The source of this chilling, penetrating fear was death.

To me, death was the cessation of life. It meant no more *me*, forever. I couldn't fathom that thought. It scared me shitless.

I would get up from my bed and go see my mother, who liked to stay up late watching old movies. She would ask what was wrong, and in return I would ask the child's question, "Mom, what happens when you die?" I don't remember if she was surprised to hear those words. Certainly, she wasn't surprised after this scenario played itself out numerous times during my childhood.

She had a soothing answer. She described a bucolic scene where a rippling brook meandered through a green meadow. She calmed me by rubbing my back and describing this serene and beautiful place. Eventually, I would go back to bed and fall asleep.

While there were many happy moments in my childhood, there were also the horrors of an alcoholic household and the cataclysmic fights between my parents that threatened to destroy the world. My world.

At some point, I stopped getting up at night to be consoled by images of pastoral serenity. But I never stopped having the waves of terror. They were fewer and less frequent as I grew up, went away to college, joined the Peace Corps, and tried to find myself during a tumultuous time, but by then they were like smoldering embers deep within me that could flare up in the dead of night.

When I received the call from my urologist, whom we'll call Dr. Uro, I expected to receive the results of a CT scan that had been ordered due to the presence of blood in my urine. There were also trace amounts of abnormal blood cells. From our earliest days, everyone in my family – my mom, dad, and two brothers – had experienced test results that showed blood in our urine. Despite exhaustive tests, nobody had ever figured out why.

The worst procedures were performed on my brother, Dave, who was forced to go through unimaginably scary tests for a child. A tube was stuck up the part of the anatomy from which the bloody urine emanated. He was also forced to take medication that gave him pimples, made him fat and prevented him from playing sports, which were the center of our lives at the time. The doctors thought he might have a disease called nephritis, and we all worried that Dave's kidneys would stop working someday. They did – when he died in 2007 from lung cancer.

Dr. Uro was agitated as he told me he had just reviewed the results of my CT scan. It showed spots on several organs, including my kidneys, liver, pancreas, and lungs. He didn't know what they were, but he was "very concerned". On the surface, at least, this condition had nothing to do with the blood in my urine, and we needed to proceed with biopsies on these spots as soon as possible.

The wave of fear didn't hit me then. I was numb. I rose from the couch in our small sun room and walked into the living room, where my wife, Elvira, was waiting to hear the results of the conversation. She had heard enough to know it was not good news. I sat down next to her and told her what the doctor had said. She became just as numb as we stared at each other, uncomprehending.

That was the beginning. Elvira and I took a long drive and ended up in Ojai, where we split a tuna sandwich at Jersey Mike's. We couldn't believe this was happening, that our lives had suddenly changed so dramatically. Dr. Uro had found cysts on my kidneys during my annual urological exam, and it was only to prove that they were benign that he had ordered the CT scan. While these tests were conducted, I was exhibiting other symptoms, though at the time they seemed part-and-parcel of being a sixty-four-year-old man. I had a persistent queasiness, an off-and-on pain in my side, a lump under my arm that had been dismissed by a doctor as a fatty cyst, and symptoms consistent with irritable bowel syndrome. These aches and pains were annoying – just as my diagnosis a few months earlier with degenerative disc disease had been – but had not been severe enough to warrant too much concern at the time.

We did not address the implications of what we had just learned. The diagnosis was inevitable, but we did not say the words. All we knew was that we needed a plan, and we couldn't devise a plan until we knew more. We both had moments of clarity that penetrated our shock. For me, those moments revived the old terror, and a deep, hollow chill would begin in my stomach and radiate throughout my body.

We went home, looking for distractions. We caught each other's eye occasionally. Sometimes we just sighed. Sometimes, we hugged like we would never be able to hug again, and sometimes there were tears. We talked about our favorite books and decided to read those again when we had time. We decided that each night we would either watch a movie from our DVD collection or the Dodgers on TV, where we could vent frustration as they bungled their way to mediocrity.

That night, with no Dodger game, we randomly

selected *Air Force One* as our movie to watch. We were exhausted and watched it for about an hour before turning out the lights. Unfortunately, however, turning out the lights did not turn off our brains, which continued to process the events of the day, no matter how much we tried to stop them. After five minutes, the lights were back on, and we watched the end of the movie.

At 4 a.m., I awoke with a fear so deep and pervasive that I don't know what I would have done if Elvira had not been there. Maybe jumped on my bike and ridden as fast as I could in the early morning darkness. Maybe screamed obscenities until I was hoarse. Maybe slammed my fist into a wall. But Elvira *was* there, and her warmth was my comfort. The look of bedraggled no-sleep on her pretty, kind face was my assurance that whatever happened, I was not alone.

When we woke the next morning, we hoped to see in each other's eyes evidence that it had all been a bad dream, a shared nightmare that would end with the bright morning sunshine. But it was not a nightmare, and dealing with our frazzled emotions was not our only challenge. We were suddenly faced with a medical bureaucracy intent on adding insult to illness.

The first step in fleshing out my diagnosis was a CT guided biopsy, which would determine whether or not my cysts, or spots, were malignant. Because Dr. Uro had discovered the spots, the responsibility of ordering the test fell to his staffer, but she couldn't act without a referral from the Physician's Assistant.

The staffer called to say that my PA didn't have an opening for five days and I would need to wait at least a week to get a referral. This was an unacceptable delay. Elvira and I drove immediately to the PA's office and spoke with the front desk person. About three o'clock that afternoon, the PA called to say that she was very sorry to hear about my condition and would consult immediately with an oncologist.

Even though I had the feeling I might be losing all my hair in the near future, I went to get a haircut. While I was out, Elvira called her good friend, Simran, and told her what was happening. Apparently, crying was involved. The only person I had told was my older brother, Steve, who did not live locally but invited me to call him at any time for an emotion dump. Crying may have been involved here as well. We had not told anyone else, including our boys, Michael and Brian. We needed to know more.

Elvira and I took a long walk at Hendry's Beach. It was partly cloudy and a little breezy, but the sun glimmered off the ocean and small waves lapped onto shore in their regular rhythm. We talked little during the hour-and-a-half walk. During that time, the PA called, though neither of us heard the phone ring. She left a message, saying she had not been able to reach the oncologist. She was off the next day, but would submit the request for the biopsy and leave instructions for her staff to follow up.

That night, we watched part of the Dodger game and two *Seinfeld* episodes before switching to another of our classic DVDs. The movie ended at ten o'clock when for the first time in our lives we took an over-the-counter sleep aid. It helped me until about 5 a.m. but did not help Elvira; in fact, it might have had the opposite effect.

THE DIAGNOSIS NOBODY WANTS

After a joint 60 years dealing with university bureaucracy, Elvira and I retired from the University of California, Santa Barbara in 2013. The fact that organizational effectiveness depended on good communication had been proven to us many times. We also knew bad communication when we saw it, and we saw a lot of it over the next few days.

Dr. Uro's staff and the PA's staff seemed to be working at cross purposes, and I was caught in the middle. The bossy, uncompassionate assistant in Dr. Uro's office kept calling me to tell me what was necessary to get the CT biopsy scheduled, but she did nothing herself. She seemed to expect me to make the arrangements, even though the world of oncologists and radiologists was foreign to me. When she called me to ask for the fax number at my PA's office, which she easily could have looked up herself, the fury that had been building up since we received the bad news came spewing out like hot lava.

I had never yelled at a medical or any other assistant but made up for it now, telling her to shut up and listen to what I was saying. If Dr. Uro insisted on her being lead, she needed to call all these doctor's offices herself. It was *her* job, not mine, to navigate through the medical bureaucracy. If she didn't know how to do it, she needed to get out of the way and let someone else do it, because I was tired of waiting for her to act.

I'm sure I made a lifelong enemy by talking to her like that, but I didn't care. I was angry and waiting for a diagnosis was torturous. My mind gravitated to the worst-case scenario, always including cancer, inasmuch as spots on multiple organs could hardly be explained any other way. Still, I had other symptoms, and maybe the spots were a weird manifestation of something less terrible, less deadly. We hoped for a fairyland explanation even as the contours of our new reality seeped into our consciousness.

Finally, there was movement. The CT biopsy got scheduled for the following week, and Elvira and I decided that it was time to tell more people that I was sick. We asked Michael and Brian to come over, but we scared them so much by refusing to tell them why we wanted to see them that they were upset from the start. Emotions erupted, and the lack of detail about my condition provided the battlefield. There was more yelling and screaming than crying, and it was an awful night.

Elvira told her brothers; I updated mine. We told her mother, Aurora, a strong and intuitive woman who somehow already knew that something was wrong. She told me I had been a good husband and father, making me smile despite the circumstances.

We had been transported into a different life. Where Elvira and I had formerly gone on bike rides, long walks, golf outings, or dinners with friends – all the advantages of retirement – now there were blood draws, a CT guided biopsy, the excision and biopsy of a lump on my chest, an additional CT scan on my lungs, and incessant phone calls with medical personnel. Finally, the results of the biopsy came in. Dr. Uro, who had submitted the order, called.

"It's melanoma," he said.

"What?"

"Melanoma."

"Say it again."

"Mel-a-nom-a. Skin cancer."

I shared a look of incredulity with Elvira, who could hear on speaker.

"What stage?" I mumbled.

"Stage 4."

After some additional remarks, we hung up.

"This makes no sense," Elvira said angrily.

I agreed.

"We need to get another opinion."

"Definitely."

Maybe we were in denial, but the diagnosis was

insane. It sounds lame even to say it, but I always wore sunscreen. I wore a hat when I went into the sun, and I never had anything that looked like skin cancer. How could I have Stage 4 melanoma when I had played by the rules and had not the slightest hint anything was wrong until the past month or so? Did I have a terrible sunburn one summer day, or a series of terrible sunburns when I was a child before sunscreen was popular? Had I forgotten to wear my hat too often when I was living on the southern edge of the Sahara Desert for those two Peace Corps years? Had I spent too much time in Riverside walking from one end of the sun-scorched UC campus to the other?

All were possible, but guessing as to when I had my worst sunburn would not explain my melanoma. The whole thing made no sense, no sense at all.

DISTRACTIONS

I grew up in a town called Monrovia in the San Gabriel Valley. Located about five miles from my parents' house was the City of Hope, one of the nation's leading cancer treatment and research centers. In the 1960s cancer treatment was in its infancy. The people we knew who had cancer did not live very long. Being diagnosed with cancer seemed a death sentence, which was why in our youthful irreverence we called this center the City of No Hope.

Like many people growing up in the Sixties, I developed a healthy skepticism toward most of society's iconic structures. The most reviled of all these institutions was the so-called military-industrial complex, fueling the war in Vietnam along with a misguided foreign policy called the "Domino Theory". This theory held that Communism would gradually spread throughout Asia by knocking over countries one-by-one like dominoes. Other societal mainstays, such as the money-grubbing business world, nit-picky legal profession, and self-important traditional religions were all contaminated by the stink of ersatz propriety and decency. Power to the people!

In reality, however, I was not a radical, nor was I a hippie, though I did let my hair grow long in college. While I was not convinced that all American institutions were evil, I was part of a generation that questioned the role of these institutions in society and their effect on our lives. I studied literature in college because past and current writers addressed many of the same questions about life that my friends and I were asking. With respect to religion, I was totally bummed out at the age of ten by a Monsignor who told me I was going to hell if I didn't start going to church every Sunday. I walked away from church that day and didn't return until my grandfather's service years later.

During this time, I developed a spirituality that was not based in any institution or dogma. It seemed that many people from my generation, and subsequent generations for that matter, no longer thought a church, synagogue or mosque was necessary to have a personal relationship with God. On the other hand, I did not disdain those who stuck with their house of worship or found a new one.

Who was I to say whether they were right or wrong? Essentially, I thought that everyone who believed was right, and any discrepancies would get ironed out on a different plane. The only wrong thing, in my opinion, was to fight about it or kill on behalf of a religion. My heroes included Jesus Christ, Mahatma Gandhi, and John Wooden.

I realize that this belief system could be viewed as inconsistent with my fear of death, but that inconsistency did not bother me because it reminded me of my pious Catholic grandmother. Maria refused to go quietly into That Good Night even after she broke her hip at the age of 99. She was walking again by the time she was 100 and lived to be 102, kicking and fighting against the climactic event that would allow her to enter the kingdom of heaven in which she believed so deeply.

As Elvira and I tried to get from one day to the next, my PA called because she had learned of my diagnosis. She had no explanation but did have information on next steps. She had made an appointment for the following Thursday with the chair of the oncology department at Sansum Clinic. At the time, I didn't realize what a coup this was, but I found out later that people in my situation could wait much longer to get in to see any oncologist, not to mention the department chair. Thinking ahead once again, the PA had also arranged for a CT scan of my upper lungs and an exam of the bumps on my arm, chest, and back by a dermatologist.

This news made the next few days easier. We had separate visits from Elvira's RN sister-in-law,

Kim, and her brother, Gilbert. Kim shook her head at my diagnosis. It was crazy, she said. We agreed. There was no evidence that I'd ever had a cancerous spot on my skin. I'd been seeing Dr. Dermo, a dermatologist, annually for five years or so; he had frozen off some spots, but he had never spotted anything even approaching those horrible pictures of skin cancer in his office. We talked it through with Kim but came to no conclusions. We did get insights into medical matters such as possible prescription medication to settle my stomach. I had been feeling nauseated for more than a month and had lost ten pounds off my already slender frame.

Gilbert came over on Saturday to put up the blinds that had been sitting under our bed for two months and to talk about everything from the upcoming primary election to family dynamics. Gilbert had joined Elvira and her other brother, Geronimo, in spending nights sleeping on the couch at their mother's house. At the age of 91, Aurora lived very capably on her own, but she had fallen four months earlier and lay on her kitchen floor all night, her emergency alert mechanism hanging helplessly from a hook above her. Elvira and I found her the next day and took her to the hospital, where her blood pressure bottomed out at something like 62/24. She spent four days in the hospital and three weeks at a rehab facility before coming home again, but no longer spent the night alone.

While Elvira had spent the most nights at Aurora's house, Gilbert and Geronimo had both stepped up and done their share, even though they were both still working (unlike us). Now, however,

Elvira was staying home with me at night and only visited her mother during the day. Gilbert and Geronimo had recruited Michael and Brian to spend nights there as well, and everyone helped as much as they could.

As for the rest of the weekend, distractions were not just important; they were essential. In addition to our walks, car rides, books, movies, and Dodger games on TV, we tried to get creative: miniature golf, TV Land reruns for me, *Grey's Anatomy* for Elvira, and other silly activities. Nothing was off-limits, nothing was too weird. Elvira had the idea of buying old plates at a thrift store and breaking them in a vacant lot somewhere. On a drive up to the Santa Ynez Valley, I stuck my head out the passenger window and screamed as loudly as I could. Elvira bought a pig plate and pig weather vane at El Rancho Market in Santa Ynez as retail therapy.

It helped, and it didn't help. Distractions were only useful as long as they were distracting, and then it was back to our disturbing new normal. We both broke down at different times, but always for the same reason: we were helpless to do anything except wait to learn the details of the hand we had been dealt.

On Monday morning, for better or worse, that hand became a little clearer. Dr. Dermo called to confirm that the bump on my chest was melanoma, and he wanted to see me right away. Strangely, I was unmoved – either because I never doubted its malignancy or because I was in shock again – but Elvira had a mini-meltdown at the news. Her anger erupted, not at anyone, but at this unbelievable turn of events. She was tough as they come and had experienced her share of tragedy, but she did not like this at all. She sobbed uncontrollably for five minutes, then regained her composure.

"Let's go see the damn dermatologist," she said.

We did. Dr. Dermo checked me from head to toe and found absolutely nothing that looked like the origin of my melanoma.

"What the hell, doctor?" I asked, getting right to the point.

He explained that he'd seen about 15 cases in 30 years where the origin of melanoma was not the skin. It was also possible that there had been a skin lesion that had spread before my body could overpower it. He labeled it "metastatic melanoma of unknown origin." He also mentioned that he was not an oncologist but did know that former President Jimmy Carter's brain cancer, which was metastatic melanoma, was in remission due to immunotherapy.

Not able to refrain from Googling these terms now that they had much greater relevance, Elvira and I had both turned up information on immunotherapy, a type of cancer treatment that used the body's own immune system to fight the disease. Apparently, it was the most effective new treatment for melanoma since the 1970s. While it sounded promising, we had no idea if it would apply to my type of melanoma or if it would be available. We would need to wait until my meeting with the oncologist on Thursday.

In the meantime, Dr. Onco ordered a PET scan, which ran radioactive glucose (sugar) through all my organs to determine whether or not the cancer had infiltrated them. (Cancer cells use glucose at a much faster rate than normal cells.) The prep involved a low-carb, low-sugar diet for 24 hours and fasting for six hours beforehand. The test itself had me lying inside a huge plastic tube for forty-five minutes without moving. I stumbled through the rest of the day but perked up that evening when Brian and his girlfriend Rachel brought over yellowtail that he had caught, which we roasted with rosemary potatoes and snow peas.

Next stop: Dr. Onco on Thursday.

DR. ONCO

It was the scariest moment thus far. With information gleaned from all my tests, an oncologist would come up with a full description of my disease and perhaps a prognosis. No sleep the night before for either of us, despite the drugs.

Dr. Onco walked into the office and introduced himself, sitting down immediately to get down to business. He was medium height and weight with dark hair, prominent black glasses, and a kind face. He wore a dark shirt with a bright multi-colored tie and silver tie clip.

He had my CT and PET scans up on the screen and turned it toward us so that we could see everything he saw. Pointing out which organ was which and the meaning of the bright spots and dark spots, he showed us where the melanoma had metastasized. He acknowledged that the spots were widespread on my liver, lungs and pancreas, but not concentrated anywhere except my kidney, where a huge lump protruded. Interested in his reaction as much as the details on the screen, I did not see any hint that he considered my case a lost cause. His even temperament and measured voice reminded me of the scientists I knew at the university. They analyzed and evaluated extensively before drawing any conclusions.

Dr. Onco echoed what Dr. Dermo had said about melanomas potentially starting beneath the skin with no visible lesion. The disease could have started innocently and inconspicuously many years earlier and only now erupted into a full-blown attack. In any event, he said, knowing the origin was not essential to treating the disease because the treatments would be systemic, designed to knock out the cancer everywhere it hid. He added the good news that my organs seemed to be working fine.

He looked confused when checking one of the test results on the screen and got on the phone, asking a nurse about them. After hanging up, he explained that the course of treatment would depend on whether or not a BRAF mutation was present. If it was, the best approach would be an enzyme inhibitor; if it wasn't, immunotherapy would be preferable. He sounded well-versed in the use of immunotherapy, explaining that the FDA had approved several drugs for melanoma treatment.

The nurse popped her head in a few moments

later and said that the sample had not been large enough to conduct the BRAF test. Another sample had been sent to the lab, but it would take another week to get the result.

When she closed the door, I asked if it would be possible to expedite that process. Dr. Onco said he would look into it, and I had the impression he was not pleased. However, he said there were other things we could do in the meantime. He wanted an MRI of my brain to ensure that it had not been attacked by the melanoma. He also wanted a second opinion from UCLA, known for its innovative cancer treatment. He wanted to know what a melanoma expert thought before moving forward with a plan.

All in all, Elvira and I walked out of his office feeling lighter. A professional who knew what he was doing and seemed willing to use all the resources at his disposal was on our case. He promised nothing, but he seemed to believe that my problem might not be unsolvable after all.

What more can you ask of someone trying to save your life?

HURRY UP AND WAIT

Three months earlier, we celebrated Elvira's double-thirty birthday with a catered lunch at the condo we had purchased just eleven months earlier. A group of family and friends showed up at our single floor, 1200-square-foot home and celebrated by singing an off-key but enthusiastic version of "Happy

Birthday" and clubbing a piñata that we hung from the limb of a tree. The party was also the celebration of Elvira's having reached her post-retirement goal of riding 10,000 miles before her birthday. We commemorated the achievement by placing a placard on her bike stationed outside the front door.

Some of Elvira's friends at the party were members of her craft group that had gathered for years on Monday nights at our old house in Goleta. After the boys left home, there was enough space to dedicate a room to crafting. Three or four regulars, ages sixteen to seventy, would join Elvira on Monday nights to make homemade greeting cards, felt trivets, holiday wreaths, and other items. I would do a dinner run at 7 p.m., and the most difficult part of the evening was deciding what to eat.

That was Elvira's creative outlet, enhanced and enlivened by not having to go to work five days a week, 50 weeks a year. Mine was writing. I had written one published non-fiction book, a chronicle of the Congressional campaign of a UCSB Religious Studies professor, and ten full-length works that were either unpublished or independently published by me. Seven of these were suspense novels that attempted to present a practical, peaceful path toward resolution of global conflicts. The other three were a journal of my Peace Corps adventures and young adult biographies of Albert Einstein and Charles Darwin.

Despite the fact that traditional publishers and literary agents had over the years rejected my inquiries thousands of times – literally – I kept writing. It was my creative outlet, my way of sharing my view of the world with others, even though probably only a few hundred "others" had ever read my books.

Elvira and I made no attempt to return to these activities. The world had changed too much. Even when nothing was happening with the medical establishment, we were consumed by our new circumstances. In the week before the brain MRI, I had several conversations with Dr. Onco's staffer, who was relentlessly trying to schedule my UCLA consultation. The UCLA Jonsson Comprehensive Cancer Center was one of the leading facilities in the world, and getting an appointment there was not easy. As we waited, it was as if I could feel the spots growing on my organs and the melanoma spreading throughout my body.

I became extremely impatient. I could not help but be frustrated when nothing moved, except the cancer. The Sansum Clinic staff told me that if Dr. Onco didn't get a second opinion from UCLA by June 2, there would be another two-week delay before I could meet with him.

As we waited, I had bouts of depression. The feeling that Dr. Onco had engendered with his forthright approach and can-do attitude evaporated. The logic that these things take time got lost in the emotional turmoil. I began to wonder whether this downward spiral could be stopped. Perhaps the doctors would shift the Titanic's chairs around a little, but in the end, the ship was going down.

On Wednesday evening, my feelings of helplessness became more palpable as the come-and-go pain in my side became stronger. It was in the place where, as I understood it, the mass was growing on my kidney. I took a Tylenol PM in the hope it would ease the pain and help me sleep, but it did neither. After an hour or so, unable to sleep, I rose and took a second Tylenol. No luck with that one, either. By 1 a.m., I had moved to the living room couch to give Elvira a chance to sleep. The pain was incessant, and it was impossible to get comfortable. I took an Ibuprophen and may have dozed lightly for a while before waking up and taking another one at 3 a.m. When Elvira came out to the living room to see how I was doing at 6 a.m., I had fallen into a fitful sleep but awoke immediately.

"Why don't you come back to bed?" she suggested.

I did, but it was the same story. By 8 a.m., we were up and drinking coffee, trying to decide what to do. The removal of stitches from the biopsy on my chest was scheduled for 10:30, and the brain MRI was scheduled for 12:30. We called Dr. Onco's office, and the nurse recommended going to the ER in case I had an infection. The problem was that I didn't want to miss the MRI. We decided to go to the stitch removal and see if Dr. Dermo would prescribe something for the pain in my side. The stitches were successfully removed, but Dr. Dermo did not want to prescribe pain medication without knowing what was causing the pain. He reinforced the recommendation that I go to the ER, but *after* the brain scan.

As we exited Dr. Dermo's office, I finally got my call from UCLA. Unfortunately, the call ended before I could take the number. We scurried into the waiting room, borrowed a pen and paper from the receptionist, and called the general UCLA Medical Center number. I waited anxiously on hold, but to my pleasant surprise, the first person I spoke with took my information and registered me on the spot. A few minutes later, I was transferred to the scheduling coordinator in Oncology/Dermatology. He had my referral and immediately began looking for possible appointment dates as I politely stressed the need for quick action.

"What about Tuesday or Thursday?" he said.

"Of next week?" I asked, hopefully.

"Yes, next week. We only have 20 minute slots at the moment, and a full consultation like yours will take an hour, but I think I can clear the time."

My voice shook as I said, "That would be fantastic."

Elvira and I high-fived as we walked to Radiology. I had never had an MRI, and the test turned out to be an experience in itself. There was so much pounding and banging that I could have been at a construction site. A half-hour later, I walked dizzyingly out of the MRI trailer and into the car, so that Elvira could drive us straight to the Cottage Hospital ER to see about the pain in my side.

They registered me soon after arrival, took my vitals, inserted an IV into my forearm, and sent us back into the congested waiting room with people suffering from all types of unfortunate ailments and exuding all types of nameless germs. We went in and out of the small room to get air and were called about ninety minutes later, which was not bad in our ER experience. I was taken to a back room where a very thoughtful and competent nurse asked me to estimate my pain level, which was between 7 and 8. When she asked if I would like some pain medication, I responded like a dog being offered a piece of bacon.

Because opioids can cause nausea – and I already had enough of that – the nurse administered Zofran before the pain medication. Within minutes, I felt much better.

It did not take Dr. Young – as we will call him because he was a man no older than our sons – long to appear. I was not deterred by his age, however, because both my sons are professionals and I would trust either of them with my life. The doctor had the same thoughtful demeanor as the nurse. When I summarized my experience of the past two weeks, his brow furrowed and he seemed both genuinely concerned and perhaps even intrigued by an unusual ER case. He asked a number of questions before sending me down the hall for tests.

By this time, thanks to the drugs, I might have been able to float down to the CT scan on my own, but the technician insisted I use a wheelchair. They conducted my fourth scan in two weeks and returned me to the ER, where Elvira was waiting patiently. It was another six hours before Dr. Young came in to say that there was no infection. He would take cultures, but he was confident they would be negative. He had discovered something interesting, however.

By comparing that day's CT scan with the one two weeks earlier, he found that the mass on my kidney had grown. It was now six centimeters wide instead of five. That growth could have explained my pain, and he would prescribe medication to alleviate it.

The good news was that the pain was not caused by an infection or some new condition; the bad news was that we now had proof that my kidney tumor, and by extension all my tumors, were growing as we waited for the wheels of the medical machine to grind forward. We desperately hoped for a treatment plan to emerge the following week, when appointments were scheduled with a melanoma specialist at UCLA and Dr. Onco in Santa Barbara.

UCLA

The MRI technician had told me that I might need to pick up a disk to take with me to UCLA, but I didn't understand why exactly. I called Dr. Onco's office on Friday morning and learned that the UCLA doctor would not have my brain MRI unless I picked it up at the Sansum Records Center and brought it. Inasmuch as many doctors' offices close at noon on Friday and we were planning to go down to Los Angeles on Monday, I had to hurry.

The Sansum Records Center did not look like a medical building. In fact, it was an old furniture store that had been partially remodeled. I found the address but saw no Sansum sign, only a man and a woman walking around as if lost. I parked and watched the couple approach an inconspicuous door around the side of the building. There was a canopy over the door and a doorbell, phone, and keypad on the wall beside it. The couple waited for a minute and entered, but the door was locked when I arrived.

I pressed the doorbell, but there was no response. I lifted the phone off the hook, and a woman's voice said, "I'll be with you in a minute."

A few minutes later, a short woman in very high heels appeared at the door. She invited me to follow her down a long corridor, passing numerous doors that offered no clue as to what was behind them. We must have walked almost the length of the building before reaching a set of doors with the signage "Sansum Records Office". She ushered me inside, where a man was filling out a form at a desk and a woman was sitting in the small waiting area.

It was a very strange room. It must have been 100 feet wide by 100 feet long, with no windows but plenty of artificial light. There were long rows of library-like, colored-coded shelves containing manila folders. Between the rows, there were desks with people working at computers, paying no attention to the public.

The woman handed me a form, where I indicated that I needed the results of an MRI taken the day before. She immediately left her desk and made her way through the maze to an office on the right side of the room. She stood in the doorway, speaking with someone, then returned to say she had informed her supervisor of my request. I sat in the waiting area for ten minutes before a woman emerged from an unmarked door near the supervisor's office and approached me.

"You're the one who needs the disk?"

"Yes."

"Here you are," she said, handing me a manila envelope. "It took a few minutes because I needed to download it."

"That's okay," I said.

"I also included a print-out of the report in case you need it."

I thanked her and walked out of the strange room. Once in my car, I checked to see what was in the envelope. I found a disk and a four-page report. While I didn't understand all the medical terminology, I did understand a sentence in the conclusion: "Single 10 by 8mm oval enhancing lesion in the superior aspect of the right cerebellar hemisphere most compatible with solitary metastases."

It meant I had brain cancer.

When I got home, I shared the news with Elvira. Was it a surprise to us that this rampaging disease, after having attacked so many other organs, had made its way to my brain? No, not really. Was it disturbing? Absolutely. But over the past few weeks, we had quickly become pragmatists. Yes, I had brain cancer, but the spot sounded small, and my brain seemed otherwise healthy – or at least not in any worse shape than most other sixty-four-year-old brains.

My appointment with the UCLA melanoma specialist, Dr. Mellow, was on the Tuesday after Memorial Day. We decided to drive down to Los Angeles on the holiday. Friends who lived in Tarzana had offered an extra bedroom to us. By coming down the day before my appointment, we would need to drive only 14 miles in LA traffic on Tuesday instead of close to 100 miles through rush hour traffic from Santa Barbara.

It turned out to be a very pleasant evening. Amrita and Simran were extremely hospitable, and we ate dinner while watching the Thunder-Warriors Game 7. We left early the next morning and arrived at UCLA with time to spare. We took a short tour of the campus and were struck by the difference between UCLA and UCSB. UCSB had a rural feel to it whereas UCLA was continually growing upward on its limited square footage. The campus and its Medical Plaza looked more like New York City all the time.

We entered Dr. Mellow's office on time and checked in, receiving a questionnaire that asked about my medical history for the last fifty years. As the office bustled with activity, my appointment time came and went. Eventually, the appointment coordinator came out to tell me that he had learned the authorization from my insurance company had been rejected. He apologized for the confusion, but said I needed a "one-time agreement". Without it, they would cancel my appointment. I had never heard of a one-time agreement, nor had anyone told me I needed it. The paperwork I had brought specifically stated, "SPECIAL AUTHORIZATION INSTRUCTIONS: ONCOLOGY CONSULT FOR MALIGNANT MELANOMA STAGE 4."

I told the young man that we had come down from Santa Barbara after receiving approval for this consultation with Dr. Mellow, and I did not intend to leave without seeing him. What did I need to do?

"You could pay out of pocket."

"How much?"

"Anywhere from 400 to 1,000 dollars, depending on the complexity of the case."

"Who determines the complexity of the case?"

"The doctor."

"Do you take credit cards?" I asked.

They put us back on the schedule, and 20 minutes later we were escorted into Exam Room 7. People funneled in and out of the exam rooms for another hour or so until a young African-American Resident entered to complete my background portfolio. We talked for about 15 minutes before the Resident left, and at 4 p.m., Dr. Mellow finally made his appearance.

He was a thin Anglo man of medium height wearing a patterned gray suit, yellow tie, and mono-toned saddle shoes. He spoke quickly in a strong, but understandable, Polish accent. While the Resident sat between Elvira and me on a stool, Dr. Mellow bounded onto the window ledge and placed his shoes on the base of the exam table, where he nervously shifted them and knocked them against the metal as he spoke.

After sitting in the office for three hours and almost having my appointment cancelled, Elvira and I could have reacted in any number of ways to this herky-jerky man. But he inspired confidence immediately by describing my case and the challenges that faced us. He confirmed that the spot on my cerebellum was probably melanoma, but indicated it was small and they could probably "zap" it once or twice to get rid of it. He suggested I have a full eye exam by an ophthalmologist because melanomas sometimes start behind the eye. He was thorough and articulate about every aspect of my condition.

He became really interesting when he spoke about my options for treatment. He said that I did not have the BRAF mutation, which simplified things, and proceeded to describe the different types of immunotherapy approved by the FDA in the past few years. He explained that immunotherapy did not fight the disease directly; instead, it activated the T-cells in a person's immune system to do the work. Speaking rapidly, Dr. Mellow explained that an exciting recent development was the discovery that two of the drugs, Yervoy and Opdivo, could be combined to increase effectiveness. He cautioned, however, that while these drugs were more effective when used together, the likelihood of severe side effects also increased.

"The immune system is pumped up to such a degree that it can attack not only the melanoma but also your organs and glands, like the pituitary and the thyroid. For the most part, however, any serious side effects can be counteracted with drugs like prednisone. You should also know that even if you have the side effects and need to be taken off the immunotherapy drugs, your immune system will usually keep working against the melanoma."

"Would you recommend taking the two drugs together, Doctor?" I asked.

He nodded vigorously.

"You have a very aggressive cancer," he replied. "We need to treat it as aggressively as it behaves."

We drove home to Santa Barbara, where two days later we had a follow-up meeting with Dr. Onco. We were encouraged by Dr. Mellow's information about immunotherapy, but he was not the primary physician on my case. Besides, what was eminently doable at UCLA might not be doable at Sansum Clinic. Even if it was, the cost of a treatment that combined two very expensive new drugs might not be acceptable to my insurance company. In my nervousness, a number of negative possibilities surfaced.

Dr. Onco greeted us with the same affability and professionalism as he had shown at our first meeting. He dove right into the heart of the matter, indicating that he had spoken with Dr. Mellow.

"He's very talkative, isn't he?" he said

rhetorically. He added, "Let me say that I agree with Dr. Mellow about the treatment plan. It was exactly what I had been thinking, but I wanted to be sure."

He explained how difficult it could be for the immune system to fight the melanoma because the cancer lived in the body's own cells. Immunotherapy offered the most effective way yet of identifying and killing these cancer cells. He confirmed the points Dr. Mellow had made about the advantages of using Yervoy and Opdivo together and also confirmed that the side effects could be serious, though they were usually reversible.

I asked Dr. Onco about getting approval from the insurance company. He shrugged and replied that the drugs had been approved by the FDA and therefore should be available. For most insurance companies, only the usual co-pay would be required.

I asked him the same question I'd asked Dr. Mellow, whether he would recommend the combination treatment, and he gave a similar answer.

"We need to fight the main enemy, and that's the cancer," he said thoughtfully. "If there are side effects, we deal with them, but we need to use the most powerful drugs available, and that's Yervoy and Opdivo together."

Looking at Elvira, I said, "Works for me." She nodded, and Dr. Onco began typing orders into the computer.

THE NURSE PRACTITIONER

On Monday at noon, we met with the Nurse Practitioner (a new term for me) at Sansum Clinic Oncology & Hematology. Her office was squished into the second floor of the crowded Pueblo Street facility, across the street from an immense crane that was helping construction crews build a new state-of-the-art Cancer Center. From the window by the elevator, we watched the crane lift huge metal beams over a seemingly bottomless hole in the ground.

The NP, an articulate woman in her thirties with dark hair, took us into her office, where we had to move the chairs to avoid hitting our heads on the corner of a cabinet. She provided us with a loose-leaf binder entitled "Patient Handbook: Orientation & education materials for patients at the Cancer Center of Santa Barbara with Sansum Clinic." It was extremely comprehensive and included sections on treatment, side effects and management, research and clinical trials, and supportive care programs.

After reviewing the notebook, she turned her attention to four additional pages on each of the immunotherapy drugs they planned to give me. She started with Yervoy, also known as ipilimumab. We did not understand all the jargon in the section entitled, "How this drug works," but the basic idea was that melanoma occurred when T-cells, which normally attacked cancer cells as part of the immune system, were blocked. Yervoy unblocked the T-cells, freeing the immune system to do its job.

We discovered later that it was revolutionary

research in the 1990s at UC Berkeley by a man named Jim Allison that led to the development of Yervoy. It was approved by the FDA in 2011 as a breakthrough drug for metastatic melanoma, increasing the survival rate of patients like me significantly.

The other new drug that Dr. Onco had recommended was Opdivo, also known as nivolumab, which was approved by the FDA in 2014. Yervoy and Opdivo were both effective against melanoma on their own, but they were orders of magnitude more effective when paired.

Elvira and I liked the presentation so far.

Then the NP started on the possible side effects of immunothereapy. She started slowly, talking about fatigue, diarrhea, itching, rash, nausea, vomiting, headache, and constipation. (I might have asked how one could have both diarrhea and constipation, but I already knew the answer, having alternated between them for the past two months.) We stared stoically as the NP discussed how the drugs might make me susceptible to low white blood cell count, low sodium level, joint pain, and swelling in the arms and legs.

She continued by explaining how my immune system might go a little crazy due to the intense stimulation from the drugs. She listed 25 call-your-doctor-at-once symptoms, including sudden change in eyesight, shortness of breath, the whites of the eyes turning yellow, inability to urinate, and severe muscle pain. Many of these symptoms indicated that essential organs or glands were failing and required immediate attention.

Finally, in her quiet, rhythmic voice, the NP mentioned the possibility of "immune-mediated" problems such as pneumonitis, colitis, hepatitis, nephritis, hyperthyroidism, and hypothyroidism. At that point, she stopped, having come to the end of her presentation.

It took a moment for us to realize she was done. As the NP studied us, Elvira clasped her hands in her lap while I sighed heavily. Finally, in the stuffy little room with the sounds of medical activity in the background, we spoke.

"When can we start?" Elvira asked.

A slight smile curled the NP's lips.

"Let me check." She turned around and tapped some keys at the computer.

"The approval hasn't come through yet," she said, her smile fading.

"What?" I exclaimed, louder than I intended.

"Don't worry," she said reassuringly. "The order was put in on Thursday, and it's only Monday. It can take up to five days. I'm sure we'll have the approval soon."

With a hint of tension in her voice, Elvira asked, "Will you let us know as soon as it comes through?"

"Of course," she replied, handing me the notebook. "I'm sure it will be okay."

It was glary and humid, and the sun was hidden

by wispy clouds as we emerged from the clinic. We were both thinking the same thing as we walked to the car, but did not say it. The approval would come though – it had to.

PART TWO: TREATMENT

GETTING THERE

Time hardly seemed to move as Elvira and I waited nervously for approval of the immunotherapy regimen.

On Wednesday, I had an appointment with Dr. Ophtho. The chances were low that the melanoma had started in my eye, but both Dr. Mellow and Dr. Onco suggested I get examined. It turned out that Dr. Ophtho had been checking me regularly for any evidence of abnormal cell growth there since I started seeing her four or five years earlier. This time, as in the others, the results were negative.

She seemed as relieved as I was. My relief was based in the concern about my eyes and sight, and hers was probably based in the reassurance that she had not missed anything. None of the doctors wanted to have missed something. Dr. Dermo was clearly relieved when he had *not* discovered a suspicious lesion that he missed six months or a year ago. While it was too late to do anything about it now, Dr. Uro and my PA must have also wondered if they should have recognized a symptom that they ascribed to a more innocuous cause.

We continued to wait for approval of the immunotherapy drugs, hoping against hope that the delay was not caused by problems in my eligibility to receive them. While it was often said that waiting was the most difficult part of a process, it was not true. Not getting the approval would obviously be far worse. If I didn't get it, there would be no effective battle against the rampaging melanoma, which would continue to sweep through my body unopposed as it had been doing for who knew how long. This journal would be a very short one.

On Thursday, it would be five work days since Dr. Onco had told me he was ordering the Yervoy and Opdivo regimen. A decision by the insurance company was usually received within this time frame, according to the NP. On Friday morning, before my appointment with the radiation oncologist, I called Dr. Onco's office to see what was happening. We were fearful of hearing bad news, but we learned nothing except that the nurse would be happy to check on the status of my request.

Elvira and I then went to see the radiologist. With the new Cancer Center under construction, he was located in the basement of Cottage Hospital. Dr. Radio was a young, serious Chinese-American man who sat on a stool in a small office and discussed with us the spot on my cerebellum. Because the spot was small, he did not want to use traditional radiation, which destroyed healthy cells along with the diseased ones. His suggestion was an alternative called stereotactic radiosurgery.

Dr. Radio spoke calmly as he explained that this procedure was not really surgery because there was no incision. It used radiation waves to destroy the DNA of cancer cells so that they could not reproduce, causing the tumor to shrink. The spot on my brain was small enough for this approach, which was so focused that it minimized the chances of damaging surrounding cells. These surrounding cells were mostly responsible for balance and coordination, and the less damage to them, the better.

He explained that I would be placed in a machine like that used for CT scans. They would make a full head-mask to ensure precision and use the smallest dose of radiation possible. If I agreed to pursue this treatment, which he strongly recommended, he would send me to a neurologist first to confirm that my case was appropriate for it. If that went well, the next step would be to schedule an appointment with his technician, who he said was a physicist, to make the mask. About a week later, he would do a CT scan to ensure the location of the tumor.

It sounded good. Short and sweet, if all went well.

We left Cottage Hospital feeling good about the radiation procedure but still concerned about the delay in the immunotherapy approval. I'd turned off my phone during our meeting and was disappointed to see I had no messages when I reactivated it.

What could be taking so long?

We ran errands and had lunch, returning home mid-afternoon. It was not long afterward that my phone rang. The calling number was the Oncology & Hematology Department.

After confirming my identity, the woman said, "I'm calling to tell you that your treatment has been approved."

"That's wonderful!" I shouted, turning to Elvira and giving her the thumbs-up. "YAY!!" we chanted in unison.

The woman chuckled, apparently not accustomed to such enthusiasm from Stage 4 cancer patients and their spouses. But if that was true, I wondered why not? This could be a life-saving regimen, battling a formidable enemy with a formidable weapon. Her words were the most positive, hopeful, promising statement anyone had uttered since I got sick, and considering the situation, maybe ever.

"We've scheduled you for this coming Tuesday at 11. Can you make that?"

"Of course," I replied. "Is it okay if I come three hours early just to make sure I'm not late?"

"Fifteen minutes ahead of time will be enough," she said, still amused. "We'll see you then."

"You bet your ass you will," I said, but after she'd hung up.

HENRY AND OWEN

Before news of the immunotherapy approval, it was difficult to look forward to Saturday's visit from my former colleague from the 1996 Congressional campaign, Thu Pham. Afterward, it was difficult to imagine anything more pleasant.

As a child, Thu had moved with her family from war-torn Vietnam to Los Angeles. After high school, she made the move up the coast to go to school at UC Santa Barbara, where she met Dr. Walter Capps. Although he was a Religious Studies professor, Walter taught a class titled "The Impact of the Vietnam War on American Religion and Culture," which brought in speakers with different perspectives about the controversial war. Perhaps the most emotional speakers were the soldiers who had never before spoken about their war experience. They often let their guard down in front of 800 or so predominantly anti-war students, allowing for an understanding, if not acceptance, on a human level.

After losing his campaign for Congress in the Contract with America year of 1994, Walter did not want to wait long before announcing his intention to run again. He was confident he could win in 1996, but he needed help early from staffers who might or might not get paid, depending on how much money was raised. Coincidentally, by this time, I had separated from UCSB to work on a novel. When Walter called, I said of course I'd help. In June 1995 Thu and I became the only staffers on the Walter Capps for Congress campaign, a full nine months before the primary and sixteen months before the general election.

We worked from Walter's "Carriage House," a garage converted into a study with thousands of books, several desks, a grand piano, and a tuba. After a few months, we moved into a tiny office at the back of a yoga studio a few blocks from Walter's house near downtown Santa Barbara. For almost a year, Thu and I worked out of that office. Her primary job was fundraising, and my primary job was traveling throughout the long, narrow 22nd District of California telling people that Walter intended to run again in 1996 – and this time, he was going to win. With the help of occasional volunteers, we also took phone calls, responded to invitations, sent out mailers, filed Federal Elections Committee reports, ordered lawn signs, and tried in numerous other ways to establish a presence.

In my spare time, I continued to work on my novel.

Thu and I established a bond that would turn into a lifelong friendship. When Walter won the election, she went to D.C. with him and I stayed in Santa Barbara, becoming his Director of Constituent Service. When Walter died suddenly of a heart attack in Dulles Airport nine months after taking office, Thu stayed in D.C. and became a staffer to his widow Lois Capps, who won a special election in the District. I went back to work at UCSB, but Thu and I never lost touch.

Twenty years later, I received an email from her saying she and her family were planning a visit to Santa Barbara. By this time, she had married Charles Jefferson, a direct descendent of Thomas Jefferson. Charles worked inside the Beltway while preserving his conscience – not an easy task. They were bringing their eight-year-old daughter, Caroline, and their four-year-old fraternal twins, Henry and Owen. When she had initially contacted me, I told her about the cancer diagnosis without going into detail.

They arrived on Saturday and piled out of their huge rental vehicle with the energy of a Youth Soccer League team. Henry and Owen were immediately captivated by the pigs in the small front yard of our end-unit condo. The most difficult one to miss was Hazel, a cement statue weighing upwards of 200 pounds lying curled in a sleeping position with a look of contentment on her face. All of Elvira's collected pigs had names, and the boys were introduced to a hand-painted ceramic pig named Guillermo and a Talavera planter pig named Fernando. With all the pigs to see, it took us a while just to get inside the house; once we did, it was time for lunch.

We went out to the patio, but conversation was limited due to the challenges of getting young children to eat. Caroline looked around curiously, analyzing everything about this new environment, which was so different from their home in D.C. Henry and Owen were more action-oriented. As soon as they finished their sandwiches, they jumped from their parents' knees to explore the back yard. In addition to the pigs, there were live hummingbirds flitting to and from a feeder and a variety of late spring/early summer bugs. The insects crawling over and under the stone pavers fascinated them, and Owen shouted when he came across a lizard scurrying through the foliage.

Eventually, we walked down to the complex' pool, which was empty on this cloudy day. Henry and Owen stayed on the steps except when Charles hoisted one of them onto his shoulders. Caroline was a good swimmer and much more adventurous. We made a game of throwing coins into the shallow end for her to hunt down, which she did with surprising ease. As we took turns throwing coins, Thu said that Elvira provided more details about the seriousness of my condition. She was ecstatic that I had been approved for the new drugs and wanted me to keep her posted on my status. Anything she could do, she said earnestly, making eye contact, just ask.

I couldn't say anything for a minute and was saved by the fact that Henry (or was it Owen?) had to visit the bathroom yet again.

It had been almost two decades since Walter died. It was traumatic for many of us, but the only time I remember breaking down was when I tried to tell his older daughter Lisa, a psychologist, about meeting the plane from D.C. Lois and younger daughter, Laura, were on that plane, but when they opened the nose of the C-5 Galaxy, the only item in the immense hold was a casket draped in an American flag. I was describing the scene to Lisa when I suddenly began sobbing uncontrollably.

I felt horrible breaking down in front of Walter's daughter, but she consoled me, saying that our deepest pain cannot be expressed all at once; it needs to be let out a little at a time, like steam from a tea kettle.

It was hard to believe all that happened twenty years ago, especially looking at Thu. Even after having three children, she looked exactly the same.

INTRAVENOUS JOY

My body felt awful, but my spirit was soaring. The approval of immunotherapy treatment and the visit from the Pham-Jefferson family put Elvira and me on a high. All my symptoms were still there – nausea, fatigue, insomnia, pain in the back below my rib cage on the left side, and mysterious lumps around my armpit and on my back – but I would soon be injected with the most powerful drugs available for metastatic melanoma. The idea elated not just Elvira and me, but everyone we told.

Michael came over with a delicious shepherd's pie, and we celebrated even though I could eat only a little. Brian, Rachel, my brother Steve, and Aurora were similarly excited. We all understood there were no promises, but we had turned the corner from *no chance* to *real chance*, which was an exciting difference. I sent an email note to the 20-25 additional close friends who knew about our situation.

On Tuesday, June 14, shortly before 11 a.m., we arrived at the Sansum Clinic. We checked in and were directed to the waiting room. A few minutes later, an RN named Chris, who had arms bigger than my legs, led us to a room with two easy chairs. I sat in one, and Elvira sat in the straight-backed chair on the other side of the room. There was a window to my left, a sink near Elvira, a cupboard containing medical equipment, a stool on wheels, and two pumps with electric read-outs. There was also a TV on the wall facing me, which I initially assumed to be a monitor of some sort, but turned out to be a real TV.

Chris took the stool and proceeded to set up my IV. It took him a while to implant the needle, and he explained that inserting a needle for this purpose was more challenging than for taking blood in the lab. After a little poking, he tested the connection and gave it his okay. He taped the rig to my arm and left to get the drugs, returning a few minutes later with the Opdivo pouch and a second nurse to oversee the set-up. Because the procedure took three hours and there was no reason for her to observe the whole thing, Elvira left to do her mom's laundry.

Alone in the quiet of the room, I could hear the machine burp each time a drop of Opdivo left the pouch to come cascading down the flexible plastic tube. I did not feel different as the drug entered my bloodstream, but I was thrilled to have started the regimen. After a few minutes, I began to jot down these notes so that I wouldn't forget the details of my first time.

When Chris returned, he brought a brochure

from Bristol-Myers Squibb. Before he handed it to me, he suggested I not pay too much attention to the statistics, which were conservative and based on the population of melanoma patients and not my specific case. I soon understood why he said this because the life-span predictions were dire even following the regimen. On the other hand, the brochure stated that with the Opdivo + Yervoy Regimen, "tumors shrank or disappeared completely" in 50% of patients, "tumors shrank (partial response)" in 41% of patients, and "tumors disappeared completely (complete response)" in 9% of patients.

Of course, I wanted to see higher percentages, but these numbers were far better than receiving either of the drugs on its own. Compared to the rate for tumor mitigation before immunotherapy, these numbers were astronomical.

The brochure explained how the drugs worked: "YERVOY helps increase the activity of the immune system and stimulates more of the cells that help fight cancer" and "OPDIVO allows these cells to recognize melanoma and attack it."

Chris returned, and we discussed the brochure. He told me what it was like before the recent immunotherapy drugs came along, when interferon was the standard. Patients had to be on it for a year, and it make them feel like they had the flu the whole time. Many patients never completed the regimen because they couldn't stand it, and the survival rate was much lower.

At the one hour mark, Chris returned to remove

the empty pouch and run the saline solution through to ensure all the liquid had gone through the tube. Five minutes later, he started the Yervoy pouch, which would take about ninety minutes. I started to read my book as a conversation started outside the room about the horrible tragedy at the Pulse nightclub in Orlando, Florida. The senseless shooting had left 49 dead and 53 wounded.

Elvira returned with about twenty minutes left in the pouch. She said her mother had decided to build upon the improvements we had made to the house while she was in the hospital and rehab. This was a huge development because she had not made any changes since her husband, Benny, died in 1999. She wanted new blinds for the windows and a new roof and was ready to pay for them. The explanation for her decision was that she "might as well do something useful" as she sat in the house.

I was woozy by the time the Yervoy pouch was empty and the last saline solution had run through. I leaned on Elvira as we made our way outside the clinic. We had to wait for the elevator, and in the brief moment we had to ourselves, we shared a hug.

We had started to fight back.

THE DOG DAYS

Elvira and I did little the rest of that day and the next. Thursday, however, turned out to be busy. At 9:30 a.m. Elvira's craft group friends, Alicia and Lynn, arrived with frozen dinners they had made for us to bring out as we needed. They were full meals, including hearty beef stew and brown rice with ginger peach chicken, made to go directly into the crock pot. Alicia had also made homemade cinnamon rolls.

It was a good start to the day, and we were soon off to see Dr. Park, the neurologist Dr. Radio had consulted to confirm the stereotactic radiosurgery. After posing several questions and testing the strength of my arms and legs, he had me walk one foot in front of the other in a straight line and touch my nose with my head back and eyes closed. I must have passed his field sobriety test because it took him only five minutes to agree with Dr. Radio that I was a good candidate for the procedure.

On the way home, we decided to stop by the house of another craft group member, Marie, who had made frozen dinners of her own, specifically six or seven packets of spaghetti from her Basque mother's recipe. Marie's sister, Fran, a Daughter of Charity who had gone through a bout of cancer herself, was visiting with one of her colleagues, Mary Ruth. At first, when Marie invited us in, I thought I wouldn't have much energy for a visit, but Fran was a crack-up. Dedicated to service, she maintains a very informed and worldly view of current events and speaks her mind. My early years were spent in Catholic churches, and I never met any nuns like her.

I was tired when we finally got home and remained immobile through the weekend, watching the US Open golf tournament on TV. Kim came over with her positive attitude on Saturday and reiterated Chris' advice to pay no attention to statistics associated with the effectiveness of any drug. She was certain I would be in a high success rate given my age and physical condition.

Sunday was Father's Day. Michael, Brian and Rachel came over for Elvira's chicken tacos and rice. My nausea stayed in the background, and I was able to eat a full meal, which was always an important part of Father's Day. The tone was upbeat due to the fact that I had started the drug regimen. After lunch, Michael showed pictures from his recent trip to Yosemite, which reminded us very pleasantly of our own vacations in the 1990s.

The best story was what happened when Elvira made my card. She made it digitally using pictures of us and the boys collected over the years, and she set one of these pictures in the lower left corner of the card. However, when she prepared it to print, a picture of Rosie, her sister who had died of cancer in 2001, appeared there. It was weird, but she just redid the picture in the corner and re-set it to print. Rosie appeared again. Elvira shrugged and said, "Okay then," and printed the card with Rosie in the corner.

I had numerous dreams while I was resting day and night but didn't remember most of them. I did remember one that involved driving up the coast at night and stopping where a cult had taken over a piece of property. It was not a threatening situation, but it was very odd, and I asked a man why they were there. Before he could answer, I woke up to go to the bathroom, a common occurrence because I was drinking so much water all day long to flush my system. I never did find out what that cult was doing there.

My next appointment was on June 21. We returned to the Cancer Center basement for the creation of the stereotactic radiosurgery mask. A male technician took me back to one of the treatment rooms, where a female technician waited. As I lay supine on the table, they placed my head gently into a sheet of warm, wet plastic mesh.

"It'll take about ten minutes to dry," the male technician said. "Please stay perfectly still."

Which was what I did. When that part was done, the male technician placed a smaller piece of the warm, wet plastic mesh across my forehead and another piece down my nose. He placed a third piece across my chin. These pieces were allowed to dry. Finally, the female technician placed a sheet of the mesh on my face, over the other pieces.

It felt strange, but not unpleasant due to its warmth. Breathing was easy due to the mesh, and the only difficult part was not twitching or scratching my nose.

When the mesh was dry, they put the mask together and wheeled me into the machine. From their computer behind the wall, the technicians were correlating the contours of the mask with the exact position of the tumor for delivery of the radiation. When they wheeled me out, Dr. Radio gave me the thumbs-up. He said it would take them about a week to "engineer" the mask; my procedure was scheduled in ten days.

A SURPRISING MORNING

Stomach distress had been part of my life for a couple of months now. I called it queasiness when it was an unsettled feeling and nausea when it was stronger, preventing me from eating. I took Zofran and popped ginger candies, both of which helped but did not eliminate the feeling. Queasiness and nausea were apparently something I was going to have to live with for a while.

Then, suddenly, on the morning of June 22, it disappeared. The realization was immediate when I woke up. My stomach felt fine, it was quiet and calm.

I was pleasantly surprised, and so was Elvira. It was perfect because we were planning a trip down to the Camarillo Outlets that day. We had nothing special to buy, but we had decided we needed to get out of the house. Camarillo provided numerous stores, reasonable prices, and a good Mexican restaurant for lunch.

We made the trip in the late morning, walked through 15 to 20 stores, ate lunch, and were home in the early afternoon. While we were on the road, Elvira's niece, Marina, had called to ask if she could drop by with her one-year-old baby, Sophia. Marina and Jorge lived in LA, but Marina was in town to visit her parents and knew how excited Elvira would be to see her cute and talkative niece. She came over and sat with us in for two hours in our sun room on a warm afternoon.

The next day, we had more visitors: our friends Roger and Sheryl from Riverside. Roger and I had met as student workers in the UC Riverside library, where I had managed to secure a job after my first two years at school working as a dishwasher and a janitor. It turned out to be more of an upgrade than I realized. While I had mostly daytime shifts at the beginning, I worked my way into Roger's position when he left, which was the 8 p.m. to midnight shift. He explained how the Reserve Book Room housed the library's expensive Art History books. In the evening, the Art History majors would come into the Reserve Book Room to review them. He set up a kind of tea bar behind the check-out counter and found appropriate moments to invite these young women to take a break behind the counter with a cup of herbal tea.

While Roger and I agreed that this was the best job of our lives, he did subsequently have a career as a biologist, college instructor, and study skills counselor at UCR. An articulate scientist, he walked me through the cancer treatment process I was going through. He explained how the immune system worked, especially T-cells.

As we always did when Roger and Sheryl came to visit, we went out for a nice dinner, and the conversation was more light-hearted at Le Café Stella.

Over the next few days, my first side effect from the immunotherapy drugs appeared. An itchy red rash emerged on my arms, torso, back, and groin. It was hardly noticeable at first, but each day it became redder and itchier. As side effects go, it was not bad, disruptive only of a good night's sleep.

On June 27, Elvira and I drove up the coast to Cambria, a small town of 6,000 on Highway 1 about 35 miles north of San Luis Obispo and 90 miles south of Big Sur. Cambria was the first place Elvira and I ever went away together, more than twenty years earlier. Since then, we had made stayed numerous times at the Cambria Pines Lodge and VRBOs in town. Our favorite place was a beautiful house on the rocks overlooking the ocean by Sea Otter Cove, where Elvira took me for my sixtieth birthday. Since then, we had managed to afford two other vacations at the Sea Otter house.

The temperature was in the 70s and clear as we made the two-and-a-half hour drive up the coast. We arrived hungry – my stomach still behaving – ready for our favorite meal: a tri-tip sandwich and fries at the Main Street Grill. Afterward, we drove across Highway 1 to the Fiscalini Ranch, a large preserve with winding trails overlooking the ocean. We followed the sinuous boardwalk along the inlets with strong waves crashing against the dark rocks. The colors of the water changed with every turn in the path, from deepest blue to bright seafoam green, as the waves rolled in from the southeast with the prevailing breeze.

We left the boardwalk to climb to the preserve's upper road, approximately 100 feet high. This road would take us onto the north side of Fiscalini, where we could cut through the neighborhood to Shamel Park and its bathroom.

We took the boardwalk straight back through the preserve to complete the four-mile walk. Elvira was not tested by the distance, but it was a lot of exercise for me. However, it was invigorating, not exhausting. My mind wandered as I enjoyed the natural beauty, thinking about the term "natural" and what it meant. Was what was happening to my body natural? Cells growing out of control and threatening my organs didn't sound natural, but there was nothing more natural than for people ultimately to get sick and die.

I smiled and thought of the classic movie, *Arthur*, with Dudley Moore as a multi-millionaire and John Gielgud as Hobson, his butler/surrogate father. When Hobson learns he's dying, he admits to being afraid. Eventually, however, he tells Arthur he didn't need to be afraid of death. "It's natural," he says, serenely.

RASH, RADIATION AND KOUFAX

My rash had gotten worse. It had taken hold on my torso, and the raw pinkish skin was turning into sensitive red bumps that itched at the touch of any fabric or the pressure of the back of a chair or a bed. We called Dr. Onco's office.

There was a quick call-back from the NP who had described the litany of side effects to us. Although an itchy rash could have been considered a lesser side effect, given the grievous nature of some of the others, I had no sense of trivialization. She seemed to appreciate how uncomfortable a rash could be and took appropriate action by setting up an appointment for me to see Dr. Dermo.

His usual efficient self, Dr. Dermo did a thorough exam. He took a biopsy from my back and prescribed a corticosteroid cream for relief. When he mentioned over-the-counter Benadryl as potentially helpful, I asked if he thought an antihistamine might inhibit the workings of the immunotherapy drugs. He said no, Benadryl was no problem, but I was not convinced. I was afraid of doing something that would interfere with my regimen. In an overabundance of caution, I bought the topical cream and some Benadryl, but put the Benadryl in the closet to use only if the rash got worse.

When we returned home, Elvira decided to take a bike ride. We agreed that I would meet her at Goleta Beach, where she would normally stop for a water break. Before these medical reports had disrupted our lives, we had ridden our bikes three or four times a week. We would stay together for portions of the ride, but she liked to stretch her legs further and ride faster. We would separate about halfway and meet at home, where I would make us each a big glass of sparkling cold lemon water.

After retirement, Elvira had used bike riding to reclaim her health. She lost weight and overcame her health issues at the same time as she grinded out the miles with impressive self-discipline. It was good to see her on her bike again.

The next day was radiation day, and we returned to the basement of Cottage Hospital for my stereotactic radiosurgery. This term was a misnomer because, as Dr. Radio had described, no real surgery was involved; instead, it was one strong dose of precisely targeted radiation. As we sat in the waiting room, we witnessed a traditional event. A doctor, who was also a cancer patient, came out of a room after completing his 30th and final radiation treatment. The nurses invited him to ring a victory bell by their station, hung there for this kind of celebration.

The radiosurgery process was fascinating. My job was to lie still as the technicians moved the machine's waves around my head, correlating the marks on my mask to the indicators in the computer software. The machine grunted and groaned, then whirred around my head as if excited to find the right spot to zap me. When I emerged thirty minutes later, Dr. Radio greeted me, saying everything had gone smoothly. We would learn the result in an MRI, which would be taken at the same time as a CT scan at the end of my combination immunotherapy regimen.

I thanked Dr. Radio profusely for his help, and Elvira and I walked away from Cottage Hospital with a feeling of accomplishment.

Nonetheless, at home, I soon became lazy, grumpy, and depressed. It didn't make sense because we had started the immunotherapy regimen and completed the radiation procedure. Everything seemed pointed in the right direction. The problem was, of course, that my body was still replete with cancerous tumors.

It took the visit from another baby to knock me out of my doldrums. Eloy was the eighteen-month-old son of Nicole, a former co-worker of Elvira's and an original member of the craft group, and Sergio, who worked for the City of Santa Barbara. We had met Eloy in the hospital on his first day on earth and had seen him several times since, always amazed at how fast he was growing. He had big brown eyes and a pouty lower lip, and his long, uncut hair was a dark silky brown. Elvira took him on a tour of the house, and like Henry and Owen, Eloy was immediately captivated by the animals displayed around the house. When he and Elvira emerged from the bedroom, he was carrying a stuffed pig as big as he was.

We had lunch in our dining room. When Nicole and Sergio were not feeding Eloy, we discussed my health, the status of mutual friends, their new car, and the Dodgers.

Sergio was a huge Dodgers' fan – Eloy had already been to a game or two – and was excited about how much better the team was playing. The relief pitching had improved, and slumping hitters had come alive. The team had shown an impressive resilience after a back injury sidelined their best player, Clayton Kershaw. They were winning anyway, and their prospects for the postseason suddenly seemed more promising.

My connection with the Dodgers extended all the way back to 1962, when the Dodgers moved to their new stadium in Chavez Ravine in Los Angeles. My father was driving a taxi in LA at the time. As my brothers and I got older, my mom had started to get odd jobs to help financially. Both parents applied for and were selected for jobs at Dodger Stadium, my dad as an usher and my mom in the concession stand. On 82 dates from April through September, my dad would rush home from his early morning taxi-driving job, pick up my mom, and off they would go to the stadium.

They were there when the sleek new stadium opened without water fountains, Maury Wills stole 104 bases, the Dodgers beat the Yankees in the World Series in 1963, Sandy Koufax pitched his perfect game, Don Drysdale had his 58-inning scoreless streak, and the Dodgers started setting attendance records that continue to this day.

And, the amazing thing was that my brothers and I were there, too. During the summer, we went to 25 to 30 games a year. My mom and dad would check in at 4 p.m., and we'd ride down the staff elevator, sometimes with Vin Scully, to the Loge Level where my mom was working. Fortunately, we did not need to stay by the concession stand and were allowed to roam freely through the empty stands. We descended to the Field Level, where we would wait for batting practice home run balls and stuff them in the pockets of our shorts. During the game, we would get strange looks from other fans who wondered how kids had managed to catch seven or eight fouls balls apiece. We also impressed our friends at home when we brought official National League baseballs to the sandlot for over-the-line games.

When the gates opened, Mom would always make sure we had the first Dodger Dogs off the grill.

Those experiences and memories made me a hardcore Dodger fan for life. To my great joy when I met her, Elvira was also a Dodger fan. She began her relationship with the team in the 1960s when Rosie took Elvira and her brothers to the games played by the Class A affiliate, the Santa Barbara Dodgers. Though it's hard to imagine now given the town's development, they played in a dark green wood stadium near downtown.

Elvira also took Michael to his first ball game at Chavez Ravine when she was eight months pregnant with him on a bus filled with fans trying hard to be drunk before they reached the stadium. When Elvira learned she could now take Michael and Brian to several L.A. Dodger games a year and get them as many Dodger Dogs, Cracker Jack, frozen malts, popcorn, peanuts, and nachos as they wanted, she was thrilled.

In the evening, after the visit from Nicole and Sergio, Brian and Rachel brought us dinner. Brian did the cooking as Rachel, who had previously been a yoga instructor, introduced us to relaxation yoga. While I was not as limber as Elvira, the breathing techniques and ideas on how to free the mind of stressful thoughts were very useful to me over the coming weeks.

Either because of the deliciously heavy dinner or the mind-freeing yoga, I fell asleep quickly that night and had another dream. In spite of the fact that I have zero musical talent, I was part of an orchestra performing a symphony. Inexplicably, I joined in with a guitar solo and began to sing. My performance was not only at odds with the flow of the symphony but also grotesquely off-key. Nonetheless, the other musicians kept playing, and the situation seemed normal to everyone but me.

THE LOIRE VALLEY AND DR. ONCO'S VAN

On July 4, after putting up our flag, we spent the morning watching the Tour de France, which we had viewed off-and-on for years. We were especially intrigued this morning because the Tour was passing through Angers in France's Loire Valley, where we had ridden on our vacation of a lifetime a little more than two years earlier.

"That's the castle we visited," Elvira said, as the TV coverage of the Tour showed a medieval castle.

"And that's the cathedral," I added, as the view changed.

About a year after retirement, we arranged a trip to Europe. Our four-week itinerary included Paris, the Loire Valley, Florence, Sienna, several villages in Tuscany, and Rome. We had a bike tour scheduled with a local company for the Loire Valley and were looking forward to it as a down-to-earth way to visit the French countryside.

The bike tour turned into more of a trial than we anticipated. Our tour guide, Serge, had given us written directions and homemade maps, which we used on a test ride the first day. Serge's speaking English was very good, but his written English could be confusing. It was difficult to make sense of his directions, and the maps were not precise enough. We were able to find our way back to his farmhouse, but only after taking two wrong turns.

We discussed the text that had caused us to lose our way, but Serge insisted that the difficulty lay with our interpretation.

"The directions are correct," he said with an air of finality. "You'll see when I show you the other sheets. They have been used by many riders without problems."

We were skeptical, but it was clear that Serge had no intention of changing or even reviewing his directions. He was convinced that his time-tested narrative was flawless. It was this apparent belief in his infallibility that led us to add ironic syllables to his name, making him Sergepoleon from that point forward. We would not have GPS out on the road, so the lack of clarity in the directions was worrisome, but we were in too deep to back out now.

We left the farmhouse on a cool and partly cloudy April morning, riding through a patchwork landscape: green where most crops were growing, brown where the fields were fallow, and bright yellow where colza was planted. We passed large grain elevators, water towers, and vineyards on the initial 10 or 12 miles of our journey. In the first village we entered, we saw numerous troglodyte caves that had been preserved from ancient times and were now being used as storage areas, garages, and laundry rooms.

Watching the Tour, Elvira was apparently traveling in her mind to our bike ride, just as I was.

"Remember the first time we got lost out on the road?" she asked. "Sergepoleon told us to turn at the restoration site, but all the caves were under construction."

"And we ended up in the forest."

"You mean the one with the wild boar?"

I laughed at the memory. Sergepoleon had told us jokingly that he once needed to rescue riders in the Milly Forest, *le foret de Milly*, which was so far out of the way that he could not imagine anyone else getting that lost ever again. That was exactly where we found ourselves when, after two hours of riding, we heard gunshots. We stopped at the top of an incline, trying to determine if we were heading toward them or away from them. While we listened, Elvira heard rustling in the thick bushes. She edged toward the noise. Suddenly, on the other side of a flimsy wire fence, a huge, squealing boar appeared with a group of piglets following like they were running from the butcher.

Elvira jumped back but recovered quickly to get her camera. By the time she returned to the fence, the boar had fled with her piglets, which was probably fortunate because a French boar can weigh up to 500 pounds and has razor-sharp tusks.

We finally made our way out of the forest and spent the night at a charming B&B with gracious hosts, great food, and extraordinary *organique* wine. We drank two glasses of chardonnay, two glasses of sparkling wine, and two glasses of red wine without red cheeks or any hint of a hangover.

The next morning, we rode to Chateau de Brézé, best known for the well-preserved underground fortress. Four miles from Brézé, we entered Epieds and realized we had gone the wrong way again. Muttering to ourselves, we turned around and tried to head back toward our destination for the day, Fontevraud.

Sergepoleon had told us that the road to Fontevraud was sometimes blocked due to military maneuvers in the area. It was a rare occurrence, but he wanted to mention it because they used live ammunition on these maneuvers. If the road was blocked, we were not to go forward under any circumstances. He showed us the detour on the map just in case.

After riding for only a few miles, we encountered a barrier with a big sign indicating that passage was forbidden (**INTERDIT!**) due to military maneuvers.

We had no choice but to turn back toward Brézé to find the detour. Before long, we came to another sign that read "Fontevraud 10km →". We followed that road for seven kilometers, where we found another barrier across the road with the same dire warning.

"Do you think that was the detour?" I asked.

"I hope not. Sergepoleon should have checked to see if these roads would be blocked. Didn't we pay him to provide that kind of information?"

"We paid him a lot to provide exactly that kind of information."

Elvira shook her head and mounted her bike. Before we had ridden the full 7 Ks, we saw yet another sign for Fontevraud, which had to be the detour. We took the turn and soon found ourselves on an extremely busy two-lane road at rush hour. There was no bike lane. Cars going our way roared by at 80 to 90 kilometers/hour (50 to 55 miles/hour) and had to cross the middle line to pass us. Cars coming the other way had to move to the shoulder of the road to avoid a head-on collision.

It took an hour to reach the roundabout with a turn-off for Fontevraud. We were crestfallen to see that this road was also closed – not for military maneuvers this time, but for construction.

We stopped at the edge of the roundabout and dismounted. We were frustrated and exhausted, having been on our bikes for about ten hours that day, and were left with no good options. We could continue as we were going and hope to find yet another road to Fontevraud. But we had no idea how far that other road might be or if we would have enough light to make it there. Or we could take the turn-off and try to get through the construction on our bikes. The problem with that option was that if we could not get through, we would need to come back to this spot.

As we pondered our limited options, a minivan pulled up. A young woman got out, looked us up and down, and asked in English if we needed help. After thanking her for stopping, we explained the situation. She said we could definitely *not* get through the construction. However, we could get around the construction by taking small roads through several villages to the river and coming in through the other direction.

"How many kilometers would that be?" Elvira asked.

"Oh, probably 24 or 25," she replied. Fifteen or sixteen miles.

The woman paused only a moment before saying "I could give you a ride to our winery. It would only be a few kilometers from there."

"Would you do that?" Elvira said. "That would be wonderful."

The woman wasted no time in moving the two child car seats and coming around the back to help us remove the front wheels from our bikes. She explained that she and her husband were cyclists, so she was familiar with our Gitanes.

With some difficulty, we finally helped her fit the bikes in the rear, and Elvira scrunched herself into the back seat. The woman introduced herself as Mérise and said that one time she and her husband had been caught in the rain while riding and no one stopped to help them. From that point forward, they had vowed to help riders in need.

We were the beneficiaries of that vow. She turned before the construction, following a route we never would have found on our own. When she dropped us off at the winery, we had only a short ride to Fontevraud.

Sitting on our couch two years later, I said, "That woman in the van saved our butts. I was glad you took her up on her offer."

"I didn't want to ride another 15 miles."

"Me, either."

"Not to mention the fact that we would have done another 15 trying to find our way. We'd probably still be on the road if we hadn't gone with her."

We went quiet and settled into our memories. I thought about our current situation as we faced a different kind of crisis. We needed help again. This time, our rescuer was a middle-aged oncologist offering a revolutionary melanoma treatment. The road we followed with Dr. Onco would be infinitely longer and more challenging than the one we took with Mérise, but our hope was that he would be just as successful in getting us to our destination, safe and sound.

TOO MANY YOUNG PEOPLE

On July 6, we went to the Sansum Clinic for my second combination immunotherapy treatment. The waiting room contained mostly AARP types, like me, but there always seemed to be young people there as well, in their twenties or thirties. I hoped they were the patient's family members, but it wasn't clear. There was one young woman with very short hair sitting with a man, and they looked like they could have been waiting for a table at a chic Santa Barbara restaurant instead of chemotherapy. A man in his late forties or early fifties looked perfectly healthy, but a woman about the same age looked and sounded miserable, with a sallow face and mournful tone. After a short time in the waiting room, she was taken across the street to Cottage Hospital.

We were called into Dr. Onco's office, and he greeted us with his reserved amiability. He sat down and immediately began assessing my weight and vital signs, going through them one-by-one to ensure they were within limits three weeks after the first treatment. He agreed with Dr. Dermo that my rash was likely a side effect of the immunotherapy. We should monitor it, but it did not need to interfere with the regimen.

I told him that the big lump underneath my right arm and the bumps along my spine (epidermal tumors, as he called them) seemed to have shrunk over the past three weeks. He pulled up my shirt in back and checked, nodding.

"Let's hope the others have, too," he said with a brief smile. "So far, so good,"

Making his notes in the computer, he approved me for the second treatment.

Adriane was the treatment nurse, but the nurse

from my first visit, Chris, was there as the back-up to ensure they were giving the right drugs to the right person. Elvira stayed until the process was underway and took off to visit her mother around 11 a.m. She left me an energy bar, and the nurse brought orange juice, so I was fine for the approximately three hours I needed to sit in the recliner with my feet up and a needle in my arm. Our hope was that, like last time, I would feel up to lunch afterward. This time, the needle went in easily by the bone in my wrist. They started with the saline solution and followed with the Opdivo for one hour. After another flush with saline, they would switch to Yervoy for an hour-and-a-half.

As with the first treatment, I was lethargic for the next few days. My rash seemed to get worse and was now keeping me awake at night. My arms had turned a patchy bright red, and my body and groin were peppered with red splotches. Bumps had begun to appear on my upper torso, crawling up my neck onto my face; they were ever redder and itchier than the splotches. I went ahead and used not only Dr. Dermo's prescribed lotion, but also broke out the over-the-counter Benadryl. Neither helped much.

While the rash was growing more annoying all the time, it was an indication that the immunotherapy drugs were coursing through my system. It was apparently one of those side effects that I needed to put up with for the time being. It could have been a lot worse.

Time passed without much change. Then, one morning, I woke up light-headed with an upset stomach. My rash was acting up as well, and I felt prickly as if I'd been rolling in hay. We hung out at the house all day. Around 5 p.m., I rose from my recliner and immediately felt light-headed and a little disoriented.

"What's wrong?" Elvira asked, noticing my look.

"I feel dizzy."

"Sit down for a moment."

I did. I sat still, wondering what had just happened while Elvira stared.

"Are you okay?"

"Yeah, I think so. That was strange."

"Are you still dizzy?"

"A little, but it seems to be wearing off."

"Why don't you go into the bedroom and lie down?"

"Good idea."

I walked unsteadily down the hallway to the bedroom and lay down. My head seemed to have settled more than my stomach, which apparently had been as surprised as I was by the weird sensation. I rested for a couple of hours until Michael showed up for dinner.

I was not hungry but ate some of Marie's famous spaghetti before retiring. I was able to sleep and woke up feeling better, if not entirely back to normal.

Elvira and I discussed whether or not to call the doctor and decided to see how I felt during the course of the day. I continued to feel better, so we held off calling.

The next morning, as I was preparing to join a group of friends for lunch, I was hit by another wave of dizziness. It was as strong as the original one. I sent a text telling my friends that I couldn't make the lunch, and this time we did not hesitate to call the doctor's office. Dr. Onco himself called back to say that the cause was probably swelling of the brain due to radiation. Unless it became worse than I had described, he did not think it necessitated my going to Urgent Care, but he recommended I check with the radiation oncologist.

I called Dr. Radio's office and explained my situation to the nurse, who called back in the afternoon. She had spoken with the doctor, who said he was "not too worried". They would call back on Monday to see how I was doing, but I shouldn't be overly concerned.

I tried not to be. So did Elvira.

PART THREE: GETTING SERIOUS

HOME

We were fortunate to find the condo we bought the previous year. It had a good feeling to it from the beginning and met a gratifying number of our primary qualifications for a home, given our budget. It was not luxurious, but it was comfortable with good privacy. At the time, we had no idea how important that would become for us as we spent so much time there going up and down on the metastatic melanoma roller coaster.

The unit was 1,200 square feet, but the kitchen, dining area, and living room had been merged into open space with excellent natural light. There was an enclosed patio, hallway off the main room that led to a bathroom on the right, bedroom on the left, and master bedroom with bath. Behind the unit was open space known as the swale. Doors from the master bedroom opened onto the patio area enclosed by a wall with grapevines like an Italian villa.

Elvira found it by scouring the real estate listings tenaciously over a period of several months. The properties we'd seen were disappointing, to say the least, and we were beginning to wonder which of the items on our "must have" list would need to be sacrificed. We got in early on this property, however, and our offer was accepted.

We moved into our new condo in March 2015 and quickly adapted to our quiet new home. The condo was located in a well-maintained community overlooking the length of mountains running north behind Santa Barbara. We liked every aspect of our condo, including our friendly and supportive neighbors, John and Mary. The aspects of our new home that we didn't like? It's limited ability to dispel heat during the summer and the ants that marched into our kitchen and bathrooms. Other than that, we were comfortable, and our condo felt like home.

That was sixteen months ago, when we were both healthy. At the time, I weighed 150 pounds, slender for nearly 6 feet tall but not nearly as skinny as I was now. I had enjoyed a brief respite from the nausea, but it had returned. By the end of July, there were times when I couldn't stand the sight of food, and other times when I could eat with only a modicum of distress. Most of the time, my reaction to food was somewhere in between, and I would dive into a meal only to lose my appetite after a few bites. Realizing I needed to keep up my weight and strength to withstand the immunotherapy treatments, I would force myself to eat more than I wanted because the food looked, smelled, and tasted awful.

I was taking two types of anti-nausea medication. The Zofran, which had been so helpful when I was first diagnosed, was not as effective as it had been at first. Dr. Onco had now added Ativan, which not only settled the stomach but also helped with sleep. My sleep pattern had been completely screwed up by either the disease or the immunotherapy. I would usually take the Ativan at 9 or 10 p.m. to sleep, and it would help relax me for three or four hours.

The possibility of using medical marijuana came up repeatedly, both in my mind and conversations with others. While I knew that a lot of cancer patients used it to keep their nausea in check, I wondered if there would be any negative interaction with the new immunotherapy drugs, for which there was so little history and data. I googled "immunotherapy" and "marijuana," and there were differing opinions on the subject. The idea of using a drug without knowing its potential effect made me nervous. I wanted to avoid anything that might divert the immunotherapy drugs from their all-out assault against the cancer cells.

I decided not to use medical marijuana – assuming I could have gotten it.

As for my other side effect, my rash remained alive and well. It had receded from its high point but still caused a skin irritation on my arms, legs and torso that was annoying when I tried to sleep.

Time passed slowly leading up to my third

immunotherapy treatment on July 27. I was preoccupied with finding clever ways to outwit my nausea and get some food in me. Elvira made protein shakes: peanut butter and banana with protein powder, flax-seed oil, Ensure, almond milk, and ice. They went down more easily than solid food and provided nutrients that my body desperately needed. According to my first weigh-in with Dr. Onco, I had lost ten pounds before starting the regimen. My weight was the same at the second treatment. I attributed this stability in part to Elvira's smoothies.

For evening entertainment, we watched the Dodgers. When they were not playing, we watched lighthearted movies like *Waking Ned Devine* and *Bend It Like Beckham*. We also branched out to the movie channels and were pleased at how much we liked *Brooklyn* and *Mr. Holmes*.

The date for the treatment finally arrived. We had our pre-meeting with Dr. Onco, who said my vital signs were good. In response to my question, he said the side effects could become worse following the third treatment. Each case was different, but he admitted that the regimen had to be halted in some cases due to the more serious side effects. Some patients never went back; curiously, they often continued to improve even after the drugs were discontinued.

After his explanation, Dr. Onco wrote the orders for my treatment. The fourth and final one would be scheduled for three weeks later and would be followed by a full-body CT scan and a brain MRI. If everything was stable at that point, they would proceed with single-drug treatments of Opdivo every other week until the doctors determined they were no longer necessary or useful.

Nona was my nurse this time, and she was just as efficient and caring as Chris and Adriane had been. I was barely hooked up to the IV before I was joined by a partner in the room, a lively fellow about my age He was short, medium-build, and balding with bright blue eyes and a smile usually suffusing his face. He introduced himself as Bud and launched immediately into the details of his condition.

Several years earlier, Bud had lost a lung to Valley Fever, a disease caused by a fungus that occurs in California's San Joaquin Valley and desert areas of the Southwest and Mexico. Most infected people feel as if they have a cold or the flu and sometimes get a rash, but those with compromised immune systems could become very ill.

Now Bud had cancer in his other lung.

"It's my own fault," he said with a shrug. "I took up smoking again. I know I shouldn't have, but what can you do?"

I had planned to read while getting my treatment, but talking to him was a lot more interesting. I learned not only his medical history, but about his service in the Vietnam War, the variety of jobs he'd held over the years, numerous incidents where he had gotten in trouble with his wife, and how he'd managed to buy a huge house in the Five Cities area and keep it despite the financial pressures of his illness. He laughed about all of this and was confident that the treatment he was receiving at Sansum Clinic was going to fix his lung.

Elvira returned to find us gabbing like old friends, but the treatment wiped me out, probably more than the other two.

We barely stirred from the house that Thursday and Friday. On Saturday, a former colleague from UCSB was coming to visit. Alan had moved to Oregon after retiring and, knowing my condition, had sent me a note asking if I was up for a visit.

I rose from the recliner in our living room to get ready, and I was hit by such severe dizziness that I almost fell. I righted myself as Elvira saw what was happening and rose quickly to steady me.

"Wow," was all I could say.

"Are you okay?

"I'm not sure."

"You got dizzy when you stood up?"

I nodded.

"How do you feel now?"

"Pretty shaky."

"What do you want to do?" she asked with concern.

"I think I should lie down for a few minutes."

"I'll walk you to the bedroom. Lean on me, okay?"

As we walked slowly down the hallway, the nausea suddenly kicked in, like the swell of water behind a crushing wave. I asked Elvira to bring my iPad so that I could cancel my meeting with Alan. Then we called Dr. Radio, who suggested we move up my MRI to ensure there was no fluid buildup in the spot they had radiated. It was earlier than he'd planned to check on the effects of the radiosurgery, but he wanted to play it safe.

THE FIRE TRUCK

The dizzy spells left me limp as a rag, and I only got out of bed to go into the living room and lie on the couch. Elvira went in the opposite direction, buzzing around the house cooking, cleaning, sweeping, washing, spraying ants with vinegar, and doing our grocery runs. When she wasn't busy at our house, she was running over to Aurora's to wash her clothes and get her groceries. We were both unsettled by the prospect of my having fluid on the brain but dealt with our anxiety in different ways.

The MRI was done on Thursday. Once again, it was like a construction site in my head as the machine worked above me. We went home, hoping that Dr. Radio would call before the end of the day. At 4 p.m., the call came in, and his first words were ones patients seldom hear from their doctor. He called it a "great MRI". There was no fluid in the spot, and the tumor's surface had shrunk to 3 by 3 millimeters from its original size of 8 by 10 millimeters. He also saw no evidence of new growths on my brain.

It was a fabulous report, a second sign – the first being that my epidermal tumors were smaller – that the immunotherapy drugs were working. We celebrated that night with a simple dinner and one of our favorite feel-good movies, *Babe*. We had seen the movie numerous times, but I guess my emotions were close to the surface because I kept tearing up as the animals in the movie encountered problems. If Elvira was doing the same, she didn't let on. After the movie, she wanted to watch *Chopped*, so I went into the bedroom, where I found *Going My Way* on TV. This classic film, starring Bing Crosby and Barry Fitzgerald, made me weepy in in the best of times, especially at the end when Fitzgerald is reunited with his elderly mother from Ireland. On this night, though, the tears were flowing down my cheeks, but at least it was happy blubbering.

The emotional release must have been good for me, however, because on Friday, I was not dizzy. My stomach also felt better. Elvira made great guacamole and a special chili verde sauce to put over tamales for dinner at Aurora's with Michael, and I was able to eat.

I felt even better on Saturday and decided to run errands on my own. Elvira had been doing them all lately, but I felt capable this morning. I went to the credit union, pharmacy and Trader Joe's, running into our long-time friend Mike there. He knew about my condition and was pleased to see me up and around. So was I! When I came home, Elvira and I watched

Team USA women's soccer and ate more of her delicious verde sauce with rice for lunch.

Because I had an appetite for a change and we had not enjoyed Chinese food in a long time, I offered to run out one more time and pick up dinner: General Tau's Chicken and Szechuan Strips at a restaurant on the Mesa about five miles away. Everything was going fine until my stomach suddenly began to get jumpy on the way back. By the time I arrived home, I didn't feel right. I took Zofran immediately, but it didn't help. Within ten minutes, I was in the bathroom, puking like my insides were coming out. I was there for two hours. By that time, I was cold and clammy, and Elvira was applying compresses to my neck as I sat on the rim of the bathtub. Finally, wobbly and despondent, I went to bed.

The next day, Elvira made chicken soup, invoking a homemade remedy for my stomach problems. My nausea level remained high, and I stayed in bed all morning. I was able to eat soup for lunch. It was mild and tasty, a non-confrontational meal for my empty stomach. I could feel the nutrients coursing throughout my body. Something was still not right, however. I felt as if I was traveling through another world and could not quite work myself back to the usual one. I returned to bed and closed my eyes, hoping for stability and order.

I got neither. My stomach's sneak attack occurred in the early afternoon. I barely held on to my digested chicken soup until I reached the bathroom when it came spewing out like a

Yellowstone geyser. The vehemence of the upheaval surprised me, even after the previous night. Elvira tended to me as I dared not sit any further away from the toilet than the rim of the bathtub. Between convulsions, she left me there with the compress on my neck, listening from around the corner in the living room.

Suddenly, my stomach trembled, and I leaned closer to the toilet as a convulsion took hold. It felt like a giant hand had grabbed me around the middle and squeezed me like a tube of toothpaste. An explosion occurred at both ends as I fell to the floor, my head in the toilet, retching violently and lying in my own filth.

Elvira came rushing in and held me by the shoulders until the retching finally stopped. I lay twisted on the floor, breathless and sweating.

"I should probably go to the ER."

"Ya think?"

"Would you bring me some different clothes?"

Elvira called 911 as I cleaned up, threw the clothes I'd been wearing in the trash, and waited for her to help me back to bed. I made the mistake of asking how I looked, and she replied, as if she'd been planning the remark, "You're thin as paper and make Casper look like he has a tan."

I managed a laugh.

"Thank you for your honesty."

"You like that?"

I could see she was not as calm as she was pretending, but the levity was appreciated.

Elvira left me as a fire truck as big as our condo entered our modest complex and parked by our driveway. Three large men, made larger by the equipment they were wearing, trod through the house in their boots and entered the bedroom. They took a long look at Casper lying there and got the low-down from Elvira on my condition and the events of twenty minutes earlier. The captain turned to me to ask a few questions as one of his colleagues took my vital signs and the other got on his radio. After a brief evaluation, the captain spoke to Elvira and me together.

"I don't think this is an emergency where you need to call an ambulance. It would probably just be an unnecessary expense. If you want, we can help you get him out to the car so you can take him to the ER."

Elvira and I exchanged a look.

"That sounds fine," she said. "Thank you."

Although she had no siren, Elvira drove almost as fast as an ambulance to the ER. It was very busy there, but it was only a forty-minute wait before they did the intake on me. Because the other exam rooms were full and the less serious cases were already in the hallway, they took me to the trauma room. It was set up for treatment, but also provided storage for large pieces of equipment that hung from the ceiling, contraptions on wheels pushed into the corners, closed-door cabinets of various sizes, open shelves with smaller metal and plastic items that gave no hint as to their purpose, and lots of blankets and towels.

The nurse entered and administered Zofran through the IV they'd set up during intake. She said the doctor would be in shortly, but it was two hours before a young woman with long brown hair entered with a scribe by her side. Dr. Case explained that she had discussed my lab work with the oncologist on call at Sansum, and they did not think that I was suffering a reaction to the immunotherapy drugs. My body was producing baby white blood cells that were inconsistent with that diagnosis. They were consistent, however, with gastroenteritis.

"You mean, like the stomach flu?" Elvira asked.

"Yes. We'd like to do a few more tests and get an X-ray, but we think that's it."

"Are you going to admit him?"

"Yes, I've already sent for one of the hospitalists from Sansum. It'll take a while to sort through it all, but we want to keep you here tonight."

The hospitalist's job was to oversee the admitting process to Cottage Hospital. Even though we had our diagnosis, Elvira and I realized this process would not be quick. We were fairly comfortable in the trauma room, removed from other patients and the tumult of the ER, but we had been traumatized by the revolting nature of that day's incident. It was unnerving for my body to have gone totally haywire like that. We were being told that the cause was gastroenteritis, but was that better or worse than it's being a side effect from the immunotherapy drugs? And what did getting gastroenteritis say about the status of my immune system?

Elvira asked me periodically how I felt, and I would tell her honestly that my insides felt as if they had literally been put through the ringer. The nausea had been beaten back for the moment, but I felt a disturbance in my core that was not going away so easily. Several times, a chill rippled through me and I would shake for a minute, not with cold but with helplessness. I was exhausted by the violence of the bathroom incident and horrified at how little control I had over my body.

The hospitalist, Dr. Admit, finally arrived. He was a tall, confident man who described their plan. He wanted to hydrate me for eighteen hours and test for gastroenteritis again after the hydration. Shaking his head, he warned me that I was dangerously thin and weak.

"I'm known for speaking my mind to patients," he said earnestly, making eye contact. "So, I'm telling you straight out that you need to suck it up. I'm not just talking about the gastroenteritis. We'll do what we can for you in the hospital. When you get home, you need to eat. You need to stay strong. You can't lose any more weight because your body can't take the immunotherapy treatments if you don't eat. Do you understand what I'm saying?"

I nodded. Elvira didn't say a word as Dr. Admit

left to attend to his paperwork.

It was 10 p.m. before I was finally sent upstairs to the oncology wing on the fifth floor. Three nurses went out of their way to make me comfortable and set up the hydration. My stomach was so empty by this time – Elvira's probably was, too, but she didn't say anything – I asked if there was any possibility of getting something to eat. The cafeteria was closed, but the male nurse brought me graham crackers and apple sauce from their station.

Elvira left at 11 p.m., and I was given Ativan to help me sleep. It didn't work on this night. Lying alone in the spacious room with the shades up on the windows so that I could see the lights of the city in the distance, my thoughts crept back to Dr. Admit's comments. They had been gnawing at me vaguely for hours, but it was only now that I focused on what he had said.

Who was he to tell me to suck it up? Did he think that I wasn't eating because I didn't like the taste of the food? I wasn't eating because I *couldn't* eat, plain and simple. With the dizzy spells, the nausea had become overwhelming, preventing me from doing what I desperately wanted to do. I was fighting as hard as I could every day, every time I picked up a fork. Elvira was being as creative as she could to prepare food that wouldn't come spewing back up as soon as it worked its way down my gullet. What the hell did "suck it up" mean in this context?

My adrenaline was flowing by this time, and I was wide awake. I had worked myself into a mini-tizzy over Dr. Admit's comments, but there was something besides Dr. Admit's words and tone that had gotten under my skin, and it took a few minutes of stewing before I realized what it was – his clear opinion that I was in danger.

Elvira and I were under the impression we were moving *away* from danger. I had gone through two immunotherapy treatments, and there was preliminary evidence that the miracle drugs were working. My epidermal tumors had shrunk, and the MRI had revealed no new spots on my brain. The MRI also showed that the radiation was effective against the spot on my cerebellum, which was significantly smaller.

We were encouraged by these positive signs. We felt as if we were on the upswing, waging a successful counter-offensive against the cancer. We had a long way to go, but it was a darn good start.

But while there was every reason to be encouraged, I had to face the possibility that our counter-offensive might not be as successful as we thought. I was going downhill even as the immunotherapy was working. By eating less and less over the past weeks, I had grown weaker, and my weakness was creating a threat. The first evidence of this threat was the gastroenteritis.

Dr. Admit was worried that my immune system would become so compromised that I could no longer handle the immunotherapy drugs. In other words, the drugs could work exactly as they were intended, and I could still die. I didn't appreciate the man's attitude, but he had a point.

A SECOND NIGHT

I had to call the nurse to take me for my first trip to the bathroom, and a lab worker came in at the crack of dawn to draw blood, but the rest of the night was quiet. I woke up to a bright sun shining through the room's southeast facing windows. My hydration IV dripped steadily as Elvira arrived at 9 a.m., and I told her that I felt much better with the fluids flowing through my body.

The first doctor who came in to check on me was one of the Sansum oncologists, Dr. K, a soft-spoken man in his late forties or early fifties.

"I wanted to talk to you about your fourth treatment," he said. "It's only five days away, and it's important we do everything we can to complete the series."

"I know, doctor. It's important to us, too."

"How have you been feeling?"

I did a double-take to make sure this was a real question. After all, I was lying in hospital bed with an IV in my arm following a virtual explosion of my digestive system. But Dr. K looked deadly serious.

"It's been tough, to tell the truth," I answered. "Besides the problem that landed me in the hospital, I've had dizzy spells and strong nausea that keeps me from eating or makes me throw up what I eat. I'm losing weight and don't know what to do about it."

"You're taking Zofran and Ativan?"

"Yes."

"One thing I can do is prescribe another anti-nausea drug, Reglan, to see if that helps. You can alternate taking them."

"Do you think that will help?"

"It might get you through the fourth Yervoy-Opdivo treatment."

"You think I can still do it?"

"You've lost weight, but your vitals are good, and gastroenteritis doesn't prevent you from receiving the treatment. At this point, I would recommend that we go ahead. Your regular doctor will be away next week, but I can take over on the 18th to make sure everything is okay."

"That sounds good," I said.

"You know, I was in immunotherapy research before practicing," he said modestly. "I've been watching and participating in the development of these drugs from the beginning. I can tell you for sure that getting through your fourth treatment is very important."

We talked for a few more minutes about Dr. K's background, and he left with a hand shake and encouraging smile. It seemed as if he was not sanguine about my weight loss, but was not deterred by it, either. We were pleased that he was just as determined to get me through the full Yervoy-Opdivo regimen as Dr. Onco or we were, for that matter. It would be playing it safe to cancel the fourth infusion, and nobody wanted to play it safe.

"We didn't get all dressed up for nothin'," Elvira said in her best Scottish accent.

Our immediate goal that day, however, was to get me out of the hospital. Most of the scheduled hydration had been completed, and I was able to eat a little breakfast that didn't settle badly. Before long, another of Sansum's hospitalists came in to check on me. He went through my condition and asked the nurse to take me off the hydration to avoid fluid build-up. In terms of my going home that day, he said he wanted my white blood cell to stabilize further and to get a stool sample rule out any other cause for my symptoms. To be safe, he wanted to keep me another day.

We were disappointed but not surprised. I did think the poor fellow was being awfully optimistic to think he would get a stool sample from me, given how little I had eaten lately.

Elvira spent the day there, and Michael came to visit in the afternoon. The nurses came and went, asking questions and giving me pills. I ate lunch and dinner, which were extremely bland, but the food was edible. Half of it, anyway.

I tried to watch TV after Elvira left around 9

p.m., but my mind wasn't on it. It was still on her. She had displayed her usual good humor and infectious laugh during the course of the day, but I could tell that she was worried. I didn't know if the was following the same thought process as I had last night, but when I thought about it, I realized that she was probably way ahead of me in realizing how damaging my not eating was. It must have been agonizing for her to look on as I took two bites of something and had to push it away or rushed into the bathroom to vomit ten minutes after consuming something. She was watching me waste away, my already thin body moving steadily toward emaciation.

She'd had her share of suffering. She lost her father, maternal grandmother, and sister, Rosie, within a one-year period. Thirteen years older than Elvira, Rosie was fifty-seven when she lost her battle to breast cancer.

Aurora had carried the primary burden of raising six children on little money in a tiny house in Santa Barbara, so when Elvira was a young girl, Rosie became the kinder, gentler mother figure, the one who made Elvira feel like a special person every day. She remained a continuous presence in Elvira's life even after leaving the house and beginning her independent life. She did not have children of her own, and when the boys came into Elvira' life, she became Michael and Brian's devoted Auntie Rosie.

When I joined the family, Rosie was living in Lompoc, 50 miles away; but she worked in Santa Barbara, which gave us an opportunity to see her regularly. She was quiet and subdued, but underneath her poised exterior was an adventuress. Over the years she had shaken up parts of Santa Barbara with her Fiesta dancing, and she liked to chase fire engines with their blaring sirens. She was an extremely likeable character and always keenly devoted to her little sister.

When she got sick, Elvira was heartbroken. Rosie discovered lumps in the shower one day, and before she knew it, she was a Stage 4 cancer patient. The chemo treatments were up and down, and Rosie would look fine some days, awful on others. Over the course of several years, she had lost weight and had aged, but the doctors were optimistic. Unfortunately, just when it seemed she had turned a critical corner, the disease took control. She died in Aurora's house, with one last squeeze of Elvira's hand.

NUMBER 43

Dr. K was in my hospital room bright and early the next morning. After asking me how I was feeling and reviewing the results of my latest bloodwork, he said he saw no reason to cancel the fourth immunotherapy treatment.

An hour later, the hospitalist came in to determine whether or not I could be released that day. He seemed satisfied with my lab work but disappointed that no stools had been produced to confirm the gastroenteritis diagnosis. I convinced him, however, that he might need to wait a long time if he insisted on that kind of proof. Finally, he said I could go home.

It was six days to the treatment. Our goal was to keep up the momentum provided by the hydration process. The problem, of course, was eating. With Dr. K's prescription for Reglan, I now had three anti-nausea drugs to juggle, and I did not hesitate to use them as we searched for palatable food. Elvira continued to think creatively. For instance, her chicken soup, after the gastroenteritis incident, had to be stricken from the menu, but she strained it and I was able to have the broth with chunks of bread. She made smoothies that provided nutrition and did not cause a violent reaction. We also stocked up on graham crackers and apple sauce. It was getting harder to find solid foods that I could keep down, but we kept thinking, *six more days, five more days, four more days*. We could do it.

I spent a lot of time watching TV. Reading and playing games on my iPad would have been excellent distractions, but these activities were disorienting for some reason and caused queasiness. I decided it would be better not to engage. As for this journal, I was no longer able to write up what was happening as it happened. Trying to do so made my brain fuzzy and my stomach lurch. I had to satisfy myself with jotting short, quick notes as reminders.

It was at this time that Elvira suggested I see Gayatri Heesen, a local acupuncturist who had effectively treated Elvira for severe menopausal symptoms. Except for an unexpected meeting or two around town, we had not seen Gayatri since she lost her husband, George, to cancer almost five years earlier. She had gone on to get her Doctor of Acupuncture and Oriental Medicine degree and was now also teaching and lecturing, but she was pleased that we had called to ask for help.

The idea was to treat my nausea, of course, but from our initial conversation there was more to it for Gayatri. She would address the immediate issue but wanted to deal with the body holistically. While the immunotherapy drugs were activating my immune system to fight the cancer cells, my body was awash in chemicals. My system as a whole was affected as well as each organ individually. She was confident that as she mitigated the nausea, the acupuncture sessions would also help me deal with the effects of these powerful drugs.

Gayatri was younger than me and about Elvira's height, with graying curly hair, a charming smile, and a face full of character. Her confidence was contagious. Being in her modest office off State Street downtown, it was possible to see not only the number of people who came to her for help, but the variety of conditions with which she dealt. She didn't mention it at our first meeting, but eventually she revealed that when George was diagnosed, he was given six months to live. She treated him twice weekly for six years before he passed away at the age of 56.

In addition to treating cancer patients, Gayatri saw people for chronic pain relief and helped women with fertility. We were there when a woman came in to announce that she was pregnant.

"Number 43!" Gayatri exclaimed, throwing her hands in the air.

She brought me down a short hallway and ushered me into a small room with no windows. After I removed my shoes, I lay supine on the treatment table with a pillow beneath my head and folded towels beneath my legs and either side of my body.

I thanked her for accepting my case. She donned a dismissive expression and replied that she was just repaying the favor. I looked at her quizzically.

"You gave me a drink of water in a different life."

I smiled. Gayatri believed this implicitly. Past lives were not only real to her; they had a strong influence on her current life. Through dreams, insights and visions, she had come to an understanding of the type of person she had been in previous lives and how those lives had led to her becoming a healer. In her view, all life was tied together in this way, a continuous flow without beginning or end. It was the same way she talked about the body, all parts working together and functioning as a single system. She believed in a unity and harmony of life with a calm reverence, and this approach helped me to trust her with my depleted body.

With my knees bent, she pulled my sweat pants up to the knee. She began inserting the thin needles into the acupuncture points corresponding to different organs. Apparently, there were points in my feet corresponding to nausea, and she inserted several needles that I could barely feel. She also placed at least one needle on each calf. Then she moved around and inserted several needles into each ear, which made them itch for just a second. She placed two needles on the underside of each forearm and set my hands on the folded towels.

"You doing all right?" she asked quietly.

"Fine."

"Would you like the fan on you?"

"Good idea."

"Would you like me to turn up the music?"

It was soft instrumental music with an Eastern flavor, slow and rhythmic.

"I would, yes."

She turned down the light and disappeared from the room.

I was left alone with the soft breeze wafting over my body, the music playing gently in the darkened room, and needles sticking out from my body. My only problem was that my rash was making me itch. While scratching usually made the itching worse, it was hard to ignore certain areas. I slowly moved my left arm to my right leg and scratched lightly. It felt better, but my left shoulder suddenly itched terribly, and I moved my right hand to scratch it.

Suddenly, I was itching all over. I shook my head, knowing it was a losing battle.

Stop it!

I closed my eyes. The itches were intense, and I couldn't think of anything else at first; but if I didn't scratch them, they diminished in intensity. My mind began to free up a little, and I turned my attention to the music, soft and soothing. Thoughts drifted in and out of my mind, but I brought my attention back to the melody. The buoyant sounds were so light and airy that I could almost float away on the notes as they were played, weightless and free.

That was the state in which Gayatri found me when she reappeared, opening the door quietly and turning up the light.

"How was that?" she asked.

"It was good."

"Do you want to come back?"

"Absolutely."

She smiled.

"We'll set it up."

FOURTH AND FINAL

On August 17 Elvira and I drove to Sansum Clinic for my fourth and final combination immunotherapy treatment. We met first with Dr. K, who said my bloodwork looked fine and repeated his position that neither my weight loss nor the gastroenteritis should stop us from moving forward. He walked us down to Adriane, who had been the nurse for my second visit, and we were ready to go.

This time I had no company, for which I was grateful. Between the nausea and our anxiety about my being healthy enough for my treatment, it had been a long six days following my hospital discharge. Elvira and I were exhausted but also relieved, having made it to the last combination treatment. It was a huge milestone in the regimen, and as the IV was slipped into my arm, I relaxed.

I probably could have fallen asleep then, but I waited until Elvira left to visit her mom fifteen minutes later. She gave me a fleeting smile and a high-five to my free hand, turning out the lights in the room. The unshaded window kept the room from darkening much, but it didn't matter. I leaned back in the recliner and closed my eyes, listening to the dripping of Yervoy through the plastic tube. The sound was not as rhythmic as Gayatri's music, but it was just as soothing.

My thoughts drifted to practical things – how to pay an unexpected supplemental tax bill on our condo and what to get at the grocery store if I felt up to stopping on the way home. Elvira was getting more creative all the time with my diet and had some menu ideas to share. I also thought about how well the Dodgers were doing. They had clobbered the Phillies 15-5 the previous night and were now in first place by 1½ games, thanks to the Giants' continuing collapse.

My thoughts continued to drift as Adriane came in to check on me.

"Comfortable?" she asked.

"Very."

"Need anything to drink?"

"Not right now, thanks."

She disappeared. I closed my eyes again, and this time my thoughts returned to Elvira and her sister after Rosie had squeezed her hand the final time. The service was beautiful but heart-wrenching. We went on, of course. The boys went back to school, and we went back to work. But part of Elvira's world had collapsed.

Six months later, Elvira suddenly rose from her desk in the UCSB Human Resources department and stormed into the office of the staff counselor, who was a trained therapist. She closed the door behind her and came as close as she would ever come to shouting in the office.

"I'm mad, Teri! I've had three people die in one year, and now Rosie's gone. I don't know what to do."

They talked for an hour. By the end of their conversation, Teri had started the wheels in motion for Elvira to see a counselor at Hospice Santa Barbara, a fantastic local organization that helps people deal with loss. Elvira's counselor was a woman named Joann, with whom she established a strong bond over the course of eighteen months.

It was difficult to watch Elvira dealing with so much pain, but it was clear that these sessions were helpful. It was a journey of discovery – about her relationship with Rosie and about herself – as well as a healing process. One aspect of these sessions stood out above all others, and that was no shying away from the tough parts. In their quiet conversations, these two women were in attack mode. They advanced against the pain relentlessly and fearlessly, never backing down and driving through the heart of it. It was the way Elvira did things; remarkably, Joann stayed with her every step of the way.

PART FOUR: WINNING THE BATTLE, LOSING THE WAR

HOW WE GOT HERE

Life was very different back in January, when Elvira had her double-thirty birthday party. At that time, our lives revolved around the condo, our family and friends, and our retirement activities. While the condo had been refurbished not long before we purchased it and we had done some work, there were many projects that we still wanted to tackle. After going through escrow, however, we had more energy than money. We figured it would take us at least two years, maybe more, to reorient ourselves financially and take on projects like installing a gas stove, having the driveway redone, or redoing the steeped part of the roof. In the meantime, we could putter around the house and consider smaller projects.

With respect to family and friends, we were lucky as 2016 began. Both Michael and Brian were healthy and doing well, which was not to say there were not stress points. They had both taken non-traditional routes to their careers after high school, going to college in bits and pieces and taking their time to decide what each wanted to do.

After years working in real estate, Michael had started his own company. He had the accounting skills, practical experience, and personality to succeed, but getting a business off the ground in the competitive market of Santa Barbara was difficult. Brian was working just as hard at a start-up in Goleta. He had begun at the bottom and worked his way up, combining his understanding of complex scientific concepts and the ability to design and build mechanisms for testing and implementation.

Neither job was easy, but both young men were tenacious. They worked hard and played hard. Michael was an avid surfer, skilled snowboarder, and determined dirt bike rider. Brian liked to free dive, mountain climb, and spend time restoring his 1985 Land Cruiser. Both were horrified to learn of my diagnosis, but both rose to the occasion in every way.

However, the first family crisis of 2016 was not my diagnosis. It was Aurora's fall in late January. She spent three days in the hospital and three weeks at a rehab center, after which she was not mobile enough to make her own meals or spend the night alone. Nor was she ready to manage her follow-up care by a nurse, physical therapist, occupational therapist, and others. Elvira took the lead with these efforts, spending long days and many nights at her mother's house.

As this scenario was playing out, I began to feel less than 100 percent. The first hint of a problem came when I was scrubbing hard in Aurora's kitchen. I had a sharp pain that tingled down my neck to my back. At first, I thought I was just overdoing it and eased off, but the pain persisted. Around the same time, I noticed a lump below my right underarm. It was large and soft, and it occurred to me that after all these years of baseball and basketball, I had finally torn my rotator cuff.

I made a doctor's appointment and was told that the lump was a harmless fleshy cyst. The next day the doctor called to tell me the X-rays had revealed moderate to severe degenerative disc disease and suggested physical therapy.

Over the next few weeks, other health problems emerged. I had an off-and-on pain below the rib cage on my left side. I didn't know what I had done to cause an injury there, but it wasn't serious. At the same time, however, I wasn't feeling in top shape. Elvira and I were still riding our bikes vigorously three times a week and playing golf once a week, but I was tiring more easily. My fatigue could have been attributed to the fact that I wasn't sleeping as well as I normally did, uncharacteristically waking up in the middle of the night and not being able to get back to sleep. Even more unusual was that my stomach was often testy, a queasiness that made me think twice about eating anything greasy or spicy.

The queasiness eventually became bad enough for me to wonder if I had irritable bowel syndrome, but my overall explanation for this wave of health problems was that I was sixty-four years old. I would need to adjust to my new reality; it was as simple as that.

It was around this time that I had my annual check-up with Dr. Uro, which eventually led to the diagnosis of metastatic melanoma followed by the immunotherapy regimen. The regimen was apparently helping, but the side effects were getting worse. The dizzy spells after the third treatment had caused strong nausea, but I rebounded after receiving hydration. After the fourth treatment, I was able to consume only small portions of a meal. Elvira and I continued to hunt for foods that would go down more easily, but eggs, cereal, fruit, turkey, nuts, and other foods could be consumed – and held down – only in minute quantities.

Finally, it was impossible to eat solid food without throwing up, or coming too close to it for comfort. To my dismay, I could no longer tolerate Elvira's protein shakes. We implemented what we called the "sippy-cup diet," which involved chicken broth, Miso soup, and other nutritious liquids, but no solids. I drank lots of ginger and peppermint tea, sucked endless ginger candies, and juggled my three anti-nausea medications like a circus performer.

I spent whole days lying on the bed or the couch, trying not to think negative thoughts. It was difficult. The most prevalent negative thoughts involved my brother, Dave, who like Rosie had died at age fifty-seven. He had lung cancer, though his body was so ravaged by years of neglect and abuse, it must have been hard to determine a single cause of death. He was only 363 days older than me.

It was depressing whenever I thought of Dave's sad life. In his youth, he was talented in so many ways, but he was also the most self-destructive person I've ever known. Every time he got near success, he would do something to screw it up. I suppose this behavior was not unusual given that he was the middle child in an alcoholic household, but it was exasperating to watch his talent go to waste.

As a youngster, Dave had gone through torturous testing, and as a young adult, he lived with a carelessness that belied his intelligence. He was too smart not to know what he was doing to himself as he smoked and drank to excess, and got into fight after fight. I saw him in a college game when a pitcher about 6'3" and 200 pounds launched a 90-plus mile-an-hour fastball at Dave's head. This was in 1972, before batting helmets were mandatory, and Dave wasn't wearing one. He ended up flat on his back in the batter's box, but popped up immediately and began yelling at the pitcher, "Go ahead, try it again, you sonuvabitch, go ahead, I'm here, c'mon, you chicken-shit bastard, try it again!"

Despite his talent, Dave's pride and stubbornness prevented him from making the big leagues. When he wasn't drafted, he gave up on baseball. He transitioned to golf, where he hoped to become a pro at age fifty with the Senior Tour. He lived off-and-on at my parents' house, scraping by on his bartender's pay and carousing heavily while working on his golf game. Late in his forties, he married a woman named Vicky, who was quirky but caring. He lived with Vicky and her cat for years before they moved to eastern Washington outside Spokane, where her grown children and grandchildren lived. Dave got a bartending job and worked on his golf game.

Suddenly, as I lay on the couch at home in August 2016, my body wrenched me from my memories. I had to run to the bathroom as a violent vomiting spell overtook me. While I was still in there, Elvira called Sansum. It was the weekend, and the on-call oncologist recommended taking me to the ER to get much-needed fluids and nutrients in me. When we arrived, Elvira had to help me in, and I'm sure I looked like I was on my last legs, even to her.

The nurse hooked me up to an IV, and the doctor, an older fellow this time, came in soon afterward, having already spoken to the oncologist on call at Sansum. He offered an opinion that seemed odd to me, that the diagnosis of gastroenteritis when I was admitted to the hospital earlier that month may have been premature, and that the episode then and episode now were both side effects from the immunotherapy drugs. Elvira and I didn't agree or disagree, but I don't think he was interested in our opinion, anyway. His next statement was on point, however, when he said that the goal was to settle my stomach and get some nutrients in me. To that end, he had ordered anti-nausea medicine and a steroid added to my hydration IV.

Once again, I was pleasantly surprised to learn

that my bloodwork had come back okay. There were no red flags, as there had been at my last ER visit with the baby white blood cells. There was no sign of infection, and my vitals remained solid. During the two-hour hydration session, my thoughts returned to Dave.

After a few years, his life in Washington fell apart, and he wanted to come back to stay with my mom, who now lived in a mobile home. My mom was upset at the idea, and my other brother Steve and I agreed that it was not a good plan. Because Steve was in L.A. at the time, he delivered the message. Dave told him to jump in a lake, or words to that effect, and my mom held her ground for about ten seconds before changing her mind. The result was that he did move in and never forgave any of us for opposing him. He would avoid me when I visited my mom. Once, I saw him at the complex pool, and he shot me a look of pure hatred. I would never have thought Dave could look at me like that.

Five years passed. I heard regularly – and stridently – from my mom about how miserable she was with Dave in her living room. They were both depressed, and he had increasing health problems, particularly gout. Steve and I sent her money because Dave had no health insurance. One day, she called to say that he had been admitted to the hospital with kidney failure.

I raced the 125 miles from Santa Barbara to San Dimas and found my brother in a hospital bed with a colostomy bag attached to him. It broke my heart. Dave looked up at me and without hesitation said,

"I'm glad you're here." I sat with him for two hours, and we talked about everything from the whiffle ball games we played as kids to the type of detective novels he might want to read while he was recuperating. The reality was, however, that he would not recuperate.

He did go home after several days but needed dialysis twice a week. It was not long before I got another call from my mom that he was in the hospital again, and this time the diagnosis was advanced lung cancer.

"Do you think I'm dying?" he asked, when I showed up at his bedside.

"I think you need to fight really hard," I replied, unable to keep from sobbing.

Nine years later, as I lay in the ER with Stage 4 cancer, I was not ready to ask myself the same question. I did know the feeling, however, of sliding down a steep slope in a free fall. All I could do was jam my palms and heels into the loose dirt, but the ground gave way and nothing slowed my momentum. The further I slid, the more helpless I felt, and I continued my uncontrolled slide toward the abyss.

A STEROID MOMENT

As required, Elvira set up an appointment with my oncologist as a follow-up to the ER visit. We met with him on September 1. It was my first official day on Medicare, so checking in at the reception desk took a little longer than usual. We still had plenty of time as we climbed into the rickety elevator with the other patients and made our way to the second floor, questioning as we always did why they didn't have stairs. We were greeted hospitably by the front desk staff and ushered into the waiting room. A nurse came in almost immediately to weigh me and take my blood pressure.

We returned to the waiting room and waited for the announcement that Dr. Onco was ready for us. The nurse showed us into his office and moments later he arrived, smiling in his modest way and shaking our hands.

He sat down and began to scan the computer screen, noting that I had been in the ER the previous week.

"You've had a hard time, I see."

"I haven't been able to eat solids for a long time," I said. "And now I'm throwing up liquids."

He pursed his lips and stared at the computer screen. The building could be falling down around him, and Dr. Onco would say in his reassuring voice that we needed to consider all our options and make a rational decision about how to proceed.

"Your weight is 123, which means you've lost 20 pounds since I saw you six weeks ago. Overall, you've lost thirty pounds from your original weight."

While Dr. Onco's tone did not change, his face reflected unease.

"Your vital signs are good, which means that you tolerated the fourth Yervoy-Opdivo treatment well."

"I'm not so sure, doctor," I interrupted. "The side effects are killing me."

I meant this figuratively, but he gave me a quick look. Nonetheless, his voice remained calm as he responded.

"Our job now is to stabilize your weight and get that nausea under control."

As he began to type into the computer, Elvira and I exchanged a look of relief. He had heard us, or more likely, he had seen the state I was in and intended to respond accordingly.

"I think it's wise to cancel the Opdivo treatment we had planned for next week. Instead, I want to put you on prednisone, a steroid, to minimize the side effects of the drugs. We can start you on 100 milligrams a day, which is a heavy dose, and gradually reduce the dosage by 20 milligrams every week. If all goes well, we can start you on the Opdivo in October."

While our main concern at the moment was my weight, I felt compelled to ask whether or not the immunotherapy would still work against the melanoma if we stopped the treatments for that long.

In a professorial tone, Dr Onco said, "Several studies have shown the immunotherapy drugs keep working even if the patient goes off the drugs completely. How long they work is unclear, but I don't think four or five weeks will be a problem."

He had mentioned this facet of the drugs before, but it was good to hear it applied to my case.

"Let's see," he added, consulting his computer. "We can start you on the higher dose of Opdivo alone on October 5. In the meantime, I'll arrange for you to get a hydration infusion with steroids today. I also see that we have a meeting next week to look at your CT scan."

"That's right," Elvira said.

"Have you had the scan yet?"

"Tomorrow morning."

"That will be a good indication of how well the immunotherapy is working. You're already had some good signs with the decrease in the size of your epidermal tumors and the MRI, but the scan should tell us a lot."

Elvira asked, "What should we expect, doctor?"

"It's hard to say," he replied thoughtfully, turning toward her and removing his glasses. "There are cases of complete remission, and there are cases where very little progress had been made. I imagine yours will show progress, given the indicators we just mentioned and the fact that you completed the full Yervoy-Opdivo regimen, but we really won't know until we look at the pictures."

He rose, indicating the meeting had come to an

end.

"In the meantime, let's hope the prednisone does the trick against the nausea. If you lose any more weight or have any other side effects, let me know immediately."

A BARIUM OVERSIGHT

The next day, Elvira and I showed up bright and early at Radiology, and I was shown into a treatment room. The technician confirmed I had not eaten, but when he asked if I'd drunk my barium that morning, I asked, "What barium?"

"You need barium for this exam.

"I do?"

"You didn't drink the barium?"

"No one told me about it."

He grimaced and said, "Let me check."

He went around the corner into the room with the huge CT scanner and spoke with someone. He returned carrying a paper bag.

"I'm afraid you need to drink the barium," he said, opening the bag. "There are two bottles. If you drink one now and one in an hour, you can come back and have your exam at 10:30."

It was a frustrating delay, and I opened my mouth to complain, but it wasn't this fellow's fault. I surprised Elvira by showing up so quickly in the waiting room. She sighed when I explained what happened and wanted to complain to someone as much as I did, but we left without comment and returned at 10:30 full of barium. At least, I was.

The CT scan was completed without any additional hitches. We would need to wait until our meeting with Dr. Onco on Wednesday for the results.

My assignment in the meantime was to take five 100-milligram tablets of prednisone every day for the next week. We had the prescription filled at Rite-Aid, and I began popping the steroid pills immediately.

I was able to eat half a bowl of cereal and a piece of toast for breakfast the next morning. They settled well in my stomach. Later that day, I ate a few bites of chicken and pasta for lunch. Elvira high-fived me like we had just won the lottery.

My body did react in one way. While I was not consuming much, it was more than I'd been able to eat for more than a month. My digestive system reacted immediately. Each bite elicited acid reflux of epic proportions. It was like a volcano erupting in my stomach with the lava exploding into my chest. I'd experiencing acid reflex my whole life – a family trait – but never anything like this.

We had an antidote, however. Elvira had spoken to the wife of another patient during my hydration at Sansum, and they had discussed her husband's severe acid reflux. The solution for him was papaya enzyme pills. At Elvira's urging, we bought a bottle on the way home, and now I was thrilled that we had. After my second internal explosion, I tried a pill and it immediately dulled the acid reflux reaction. The acid still burned in my chest, and I had to eat slowly and not have too much food at one time, but the papaya allowed me to eat..

On Saturday we expected two visits: Alicia and Matt with their two boys and Simran. That morning, as I was preparing to take my shower, I made the mistake of looking at myself in the mirror. I had caught glimpses of my slim frame as I lost weight but had not taken a full-mirror look. I knew about my face, of course, where the prominent feature had become my sunken eyes and sunken cheeks, but now I could see that my chest was sunken and my rib cage was fully exposed.

"My goodness," I mused.

I turned sideways and saw that the line of my body went straight up and down like a fence post. My feet looked way too big for my legs, and my knobby knees protruded grotesquely below my thighs, which were barely thicker than my calves.

Even though I would cover myself with layers that afternoon, I was extremely self-conscious. My appearance didn't matter to our visitors, except to encourage everyone to conjure ways to fatten me up, but I didn't like what I saw.

After a few days on the prednisone, I was eating

half a bowl of cereal and a piece of toast with tea for breakfast, and half a turkey sandwich with a few potato chips for lunch. For dinner, I could manage one or two of the tasty meatballs Alicia had made. It was great progress, attributable in part to the length of time since my last treatment, but clearly also due to the massive amount of prednisone I was taking.

While the steroids seemed to be working, my digestive system remained testy for more than a week. The papaya enzyme tamped down the ferocious acid reflux but could not eradicate it. The volcano would erupt in my stomach, but the lava would cool and lose its fire as it rose into my chest. My system seemed to be adapting just in time for our meeting with Dr. Onco on September 7, my sixty-fifth birthday.

THE REPORT

"Let's see what we have here," Dr. Onco said, as he turned his computer screen halfway toward us. I had the impression he would be seeing last Friday's CT scan results for the first time as we were. He seemed to have a classification system in his mind that became clear as he spoke: tumors and masses were the substantial cancerous growths that had height and weight while spots were smaller areas where the cancer had not developed into anything substantial.

"I'll show you the tumors on your spine from three months ago," he said, fiddling with the mouse. The X-ray image of my spine appeared on the screen.

Without touching the screen, Dr. Onco outlined the tumors with his pen. He moved the cursor and moved it to the lymph node beneath my right arm and used his pen again to outline the large mass.

"Now, I'll show you today's scan."

Elvira took my hand as we leaned closer to the screen.

"Here is the same area on your spine, and as you can see, it's normal." I squeezed Elvira's hand. Dr. Onco moved the cursor up and down as if trying to find the tumors from three months earlier.

When he moved to the lymph node area, he repeated, "Normal here as well. Let's move on to the other areas." He changed screens, pulling up the original image of my colon.

"You see the spots here, here, and here?" He pointed with his pen. "Those are melanoma." We nodded, and he pulled up the current scan, panning over the image with the cursor.

"I don't see any spots," he said simply.

Elvira and I sighed in relief. I looked at Dr. Onco, but he was already pulling up the old image of my leg, where he showed the location of the spots. When he pulled up the new image, he said, "Nothing here, either. Let's look at your organs."

He started with the lungs first, finding numerous spots on them in the three-month-old image. When he went to the five-day-old image, he scanned up and down several times before saying, "Nothing suspicious."

The same was true of the pancreas. We grew more excited with each revelation, but we also knew the two organs with medium to large masses were still to come: the liver and the kidney.

Dr. Onco started with the original image of the liver and methodically showed us both masses and spots. When he pulled up the new image, he scanned those same areas carefully. The original spots were gone, but the masses had not entirely disappeared.

"The masses are much smaller, but you can see that there's still some melanoma there."

He said it as if noting that the remainder of a storm was still in the area. My heart sank at the news that there was still cancer on my liver.

He went on to the kidney, probably the source of my disease and the location of the largest number of masses. Once again, the contrast between the original CT scan and the new one was dramatic. The spots that had covered the organ seemed to all be gone. The small masses were now spots, and the medium masses were much smaller. The huge mass that had caused me pain five months ago had been reduced by half.

Dr. Onco turned the screen back toward him and gave his assessment of the results.

"It's not a perfect report, but it's a very good one."

At the risk of stating the obvious, I asked, "It means the immunotherapy is working, right?" I wanted to hear it from him.

"Yes" he replied, the barest hint of a smile beginning to suffuse his face. "As I have told you, I have had cases with complete remission after the first phase of the regimen and also seen cases where there was no improvement. In your case, I would say there has been significant improvement."

"And no new growth?" Elvira asked.

"None that I could see."

"That's wonderful!" she exclaimed.

I took a deep breath but said nothing.

"Let's talk about your treatment," Dr. Onco said getting back down to business. "Have you been able to eat more with the prednisone?"

"It's been a struggle. I hadn't eaten for so long, and I threw up so many times, my whole digestive system seemed to be screwed up. The acid reflux was unbelievable, but papaya enzyme pills have helped."

"And the nausea?"

"It's better. I can eat again. Small portions, and I need to be careful what I eat, but it's definitely better than it was."

Elvira added, "If you compare what he was eating a week ago – or *not* eating – it's pretty remarkable."

"Okay," Dr. Onco said, nodding. "I'd like to keep you on the prednisone. We'll reduce the daily dose by 20 milligrams next week, so you'll take four pills a day instead of five. The following week, we'll reduce it again by 20 milligrams a day, and then we'll keep reducing it by 20 milligrams each week. By the time you return here on October 5, you should be weaned off the drug."

"I need to be weaned?"

"It's a strong drug."

He turned to the computer to summarize our visit and input the information about the prednisone. He mouthed much of it, including the part where he set our next meeting, and my first Opdivo-only treatment, four weeks away. He hit "enter" and rose to shake our hands.

"Congratulations," Dr. Onco said.

Instead of taking his hand, I pulled him toward me and gave him a big hug. He smiled shyly and hugged back.

Outside, Elvira and I had our own hug, expressing our joy and relief. I had started the regimen twelve weeks earlier. While we'd had positive signs, it was only now that we knew for sure that the immunotherapy drugs were working against the cancer. Our lives had changed dramatically in the past twenty minutes.

Elvira drove along Pueblo Street and turned right at the frontage road by the freeway. She followed the road to Las Positas and turned left. We didn't speak. We were still happy, of course, but something else was going on.

I thought about it for a minute and came to the conclusion that I wanted a perfect report. Dr. Onco had said that there were cases of complete remission, but we had not gotten that. Instead, we were told that things were much better than they had been and the drugs were working, but I still had metastatic melanoma in my body.

Elvira and I had known beforehand that a perfect report was unrealistic. We knew that a mixed report was the best we could hope for. But while a mixed report was intellectually acceptable, it was difficult to take emotionally. Our emotions wanted Dr. Onco to tell us the cancer was gone, and gone for good.

Elvira was the one to break the silence in the car.

"Are you okay?" she asked.

I told her what I had been thinking.

"I just want you to be better."

I nodded, tears welling up in my eyes.

"I guess we'll just need to settle for a little bit of happiness at a time."

She didn't take her eyes off the road as she reached over and found my arm, giving it a squeeze.

PART FIVE: THE WAY BACK

THE MONTH OF FOOD

As a powerful steroid, prednisone was frequently used to combat the side effects of cancer treatment. It was so strong that it could take over the job of the adrenal glands. Patients had to be weaned off it so that the adrenal glands could start functioning normally before the prednisone was stopped. In my case, the prednisone was being used to counteract my nausea, and the weaning would take five weeks, taking me from 110 milligrams a day to 0.

After our September 7 meeting with Dr. Onco, we stopped at Whole Foods. I had decided that my go-to item would be a flour tortilla burrito with pinto beans, rice, and sour cream. It had protein, and everything in it was organic. Elvira bought heartier food for herself with the hope that we could eventually share it.

The push-back from my digestive system

continued. When digestion stops being automatic, it can be hard work. The papaya enzymes were instrumental in reducing my body's reaction to solid foods. Progress seemed slow to me; but perhaps not, because I seemed to add a new item to the menu almost every day. During the second week, when I was taking 80 milligrams of prednisone a day, I took the big step of making a taco at home.

We bought onions and green peppers to cook with the ground turkey, and sharp cheese and cherry tomatoes. I would warm up the taco shell in the oven, place the tomatoes in the crisp shell, add cheese and mild salsa, and lastly spoon in the hot ground turkey mix. It was a backward taco with the meat in last, but it looked and smelled good to me. My first bite was my most exciting food moment in months.

In an odd way, the tendency of prednisone to cause insomnia helped with my food consumption. As I lay awake in the middle of the night, I would plan my meals for the day, integrating leftovers that we might have from the previous night or deciding to make chicken tacos for lunch as a change of pace. After a half hour to forty-five minutes, when I was sure sleep was not returning, I would quietly leave the bed to get what became known as my "pre-breakfast". At 4 a.m., I would sit at our dining table eating French toast with maple syrup or yogurt with granola, raspberries, and blueberries.

Afterward, I would retire to the study, where I would work on my journal. I had stopped for a long time, unable to do anything but jot occasional notes, but now I was thinking clearly again.

As the sun started to rise, I would get sleepy again. I would put the computer away and sneak back into bed. Elvira slept soundly in the early morning, and she never heard me. Having eaten and written, I had a feeling of satisfaction that helped me fall back asleep until we awoke around 8 a.m.

It was time for my regular breakfast, which usually entailed eggs and toast, maybe potatoes or meat if there were some left over from the previous night's dinner. Coffee tasted funny, so I had peppermint or green tea instead.

I had lunch at noon, tacos or a bean and cheese burrito, and between 3 and 4 p.m. one of Elvira's carb-infused peanut butter and banana smoothies. My goal was to pound the calories in there and see how much weight I could gain by October 5. Dinner could be anything from Marie's spaghetti to Elvira's baked chicken and potatoes. I had smaller helpings than Elvira but was usually able to eat a version of her meal.

Later in the evening, I would have ice cream on top of cookies or brownies if Elvira had baked them. If one counted the smoothie as dessert, that totaled six meals in twenty-four hours. My hope was that anyone eating that many meals in a day *must* gain weight.

Thinking so much about food elicited conversations about our favorite restaurant meals. A number of them occurred while Elvira and I had been traveling, beginning with our trip to Maui in 1994 at Longhi's in Lahaina. From our table on the second-floor terrace, we had an unobstructed view of a spectacular sunset striped with deep reds, brilliant oranges, and bright yellows. Elvira had peppered steak medallions, and I had the swordfish, grilled to perfection. Afterward, we split a chocolate soufflé for dessert.

The most memorable dinner from our trip to Europe in 2014 was at Café Procope in the Latin Quarter of Paris, where Benjamin Franklin, Napoléon Bonaparte, and many other historical figures of the 18th and 19th centuries had eaten. It was a formal restaurant, with heavy curtains, old-school sconces, cloth napkins, formal china, and thick leather chairs. We had mushroom soup followed by coq au vin, a chicken dish cooked in a red burgundy wine, mushrooms, and spices.

The other truly elegant meal we had on our trip was in Rome at Le Sorelle, where the dessert was unique. We let the waiter pick for us, and he brought a tray on which sat the frozen outer layer of a lemon, cactus fruit, kiwi, mango, and walnut. Inside was sorbet and gelato that looked and tasted like the fruit or nut of its container.

The food we ate on our trips brought back fond memories, but the last meal we had on our trip was hardly European because it was at Rome's Hard Rock Café. We'd been traveling for more than a month and missed American cooking. Elvira ordered The Texan, hickory-smoked pork with barbecue sauce, fried jalapenos and fried onions on a toasted brioche, and I had the decadent Legendary Burger with smoked bacon, cheese, onion ring, lettuce and, tomato. To drink, we had strawberry-basil lemonade.

Even though I was far from ready for a Legendary Burger, we dreamt of eating there again – at the Hard Rock Café in Hollywood, not Rome. In the meantime, because I now knew I could eat tacos, refried beans, and mole, I planned to take full advantage of Pepe's and Los Arroyos' take-out menus.

KNOCKING AROUND THE 120s

As I started to feel better, Aurora's brother, Uncle Frank, initiated a visit. It had been months since he brought his dog, Gitana, to see us. Black and white with a friendly disposition, Gitana was an Aussie-border collie mix weighing about 75 pounds. Before I got sick, I would walk her up to the More Mesa bluffs behind our house, and she would sniff to her heart's content for forty-five minutes. Our ambitions for this visit were significantly reduced: a walk through our complex, with Frank there to catch me if Gitana decided to sprint after a cat.

Aurora's younger brother, Frank, is in his eighties now and never married. His career was in the Air Force, for which he did a lot of traveling in Asia, and the Postal Service. He's a thoughtful and generous man but doesn't take crap from anybody and has a no-nonsense approach to life. He is well-read and up-to-date on world events, and he gives his opinion in colorful language that leaves no room for doubt about his position.

Gitana was a rescue who had lived on the streets. She was skittish at first, but Frank provided a home and she learned to trust him. She also learned to look forward to her Sunday walks with us at our previous location. When we moved to the condo, we were concerned that Gitana wouldn't adapt, but we needn't have worried. It was less than 100 yards to the bluffs, and once out there, it was open space just like we had in Goleta. We stayed in the complex for this visit, but Gitana didn't seem to mind – she was lively and energetic as always. We agreed to resume regular visits, and eventually I hoped to be able to go further than the boundary of our complex.

As the month unfolded, my nausea receded, and I kept eating. On our home scale, which showed a number about 2½ pounds less than Dr. Onco's office, my weight one week out from seeing the doctor was up to 126.6. By the 16th, it was 130.2, and by the 25th, it had reached its peak at 131.6. By that time, following the game plan on weaning me off the prednisone, I was taking only two pills, or 40 mg/day.

Unfortunately, at that point, the steroid reduction began to have an effect. My stomach felt different with hints of the familiar nausea reappearing. It seemed to grow stronger each day and was soon affecting how much I could eat.

There were other indicators of a change in my condition. First, I was tired almost all the time. Also, while my skin was rash-free, it was frequently itchy. One day, my ankles itched when I took off my socks, and I scratched my ankles satisfyingly for a minute before they became inflamed like I'd lit a fire inside there with my fingernails. I hopped around a little like I'd walked on coals and reminded myself that scratching was not my friend.

Around that same time, I noticed that my ankles were slightly swollen. I didn't pay much attention, but the next day the swelling was worse. I called Dr. Onco's office and was offered Lasix, a diuretic. I refused at first, not wanting to take any more medication than was necessary, but the next day my ankles were so fat and ugly that I called back and got started on the Lasix.

Dr. Onco attributed the edema to the prednisone, though it was odd that my ankles were swelling up as I was reducing my dosage. Maybe it was a cumulative effect. What did make sense was that the reduction in prednisone led to better sleep. I would get up during the night for shorter periods now, and sometimes not at all. I didn't miss the pre-breakfast and wasn't nearly as hungry for breakfast, either.

The date for my check-up with Dr. Onco, when he would determine whether I was fit to begin the next phase of the regimen, was approaching. I knew that I had been backsliding, no longer eating enough to sustain my weight, so I began to take the anti-nausea drugs again. With all the drugs inside me, I no longer knew what was happening with my body. I needed to take steroids to combat the side effects of the immunotherapy drugs, but the steroids also had side effects, causing me to take more drugs that could also have side effects. I was caught in a vicious cycle, and I was afraid the doctor would determine that my body simply couldn't handle more immunotherapy treatments, that we would need to put them on hold, potentially giving the cancer a chance to reassert itself.

In the meantime, the Dodgers' season was coming to a close. They were going to the playoffs and would meet the Washington Nationals in the first round. We watched and listened to Vin Scully's last games with sadness, knowing how much we would miss his unique style of calling a ball game.

On September 26, we watched the first of the Presidential Debates between Hillary Clinton and Donald Trump. We knew we wouldn't learn anything new about either of the candidates, but we watched, anyway.

It became extremely hot in Santa Barbara, the temperature rising to a record 105. We took drives in the afternoon just to take advantage of the car's air conditioning. Sleep became almost as difficult as it had been while I was taking prednisone, and Elvira was just as uncomfortable. It was 90 degrees when Elvira took me to see Gayatri on Friday September 30, five days before my meeting with Dr. Onco. At the beginning of the session, Gayatri asked how I was feeling, and I replied, "Okay." She picked up on the tone and asked, "What's up?"

If you can't be honest with your acupuncturist, who can you be honest with? I explained that the nausea had returned, and I felt tired and frustrated. In a soft voice, she told me a story.

"When George died, my grief was so heavy that

it was like walking with a bag of large stones. For a long time, I looked for a place to put the stones. I desperately wanted to rid myself of them and be free of my grief. Then I realized that I needed to keep the stones, that they were part of my journey. I needed to accept them and see the bigger purpose because carrying them was the only way to get through the grief. Once I stopped trying to rid myself of the stones and accepted them as part of me instead of a burden I was carrying, I felt free of their weight."

She exited the room and left me to ponder how I was handling the stones in my life.

At the tail end of the heat wave, Nicole and Sergio brought Eloy over for a dip in the pool. Nicole was the only adult who immersed herself, taking the eighteen-month-old on trips from one side of the pool to the other. He kicked wildly and flailed his arms trying to mimic Nicole's swim stroke. It would not be long before he was swimming on his own.

Sunday, October 2, was the last day of baseball season and the last day for Vin Scully. Between pitches, he allowed himself a few stories about himself, calling himself the skinny red-headed kid with the great opportunity to do what he loved sixty-seven years. Two months later, he would receive the Presidential Medal of Freedom.

VAPING

"One hundred twenty-nine pounds," Dr Onco

said, matter-of-factly. "A gain of six pounds in four weeks."

"It was more at one point, at least according to our home scale."

"Why is that?"

"My stomach started acting up again, and I wasn't able to eat as much."

Dr. Onco pursed his lips.

"Six pounds still means we're headed in the right direction. Your vitals are good. Cholesterol is a little high at 205. The tests have not come in yet for the pituitary and adrenal glands. They were underperforming on September 7, but that was just six days after you started the prednisone. We'll need to check on that next time, though. All in all, I think we're ready to move forward. What do you say?"

"I want to go ahead with the treatment."

With a quick glance at Elvira, he began entering the information into the computer while explaining that they would be administering a higher dose of Opdivo than before. Patients were usually able to tolerate it without major side effects. If I had any problems, however, we were to let him know immediately. He rose and shook both of our hands, indicating our meeting was over. Betsy, a nurse I had not met, found us a few minutes later in the waiting room.

After the treatment, which lasted only an hour

for the single drug, we went to breakfast, where I ordered bacon and eggs. I ate half before petering out and put the rest in a take-away box. At home, I took a long nap but was still tired and feeling out of sorts the rest of the day. We had sandwiches for dinner, but they had little flavor. I seemed to have little sense of smell or taste, and my stomach was fluttering wildly whenever I sent anything through my digestive system. The next day was just as bad, and I woke up on Friday feeling like anything I ate would come right back up.

Frustrated, I went out to our patio.

"Dammit!" I said under my breath. "Dammit, dammit, dammit!"

Elvira appeared at the screen door.

"What's wrong?"

"Oh, nothing," I said with a sigh. "It's just this stupid nausea."

"Is it bad?"

"Not as bad as the sippy-cup days, but bad enough. I need to be able to eat."

"I know," she said, coming onto the patio and draping any arm around my shoulder.

"Onco said the side effects wouldn't be so bad with the single drug. You coulda fooled me."

"Did you take a Zofran?"

Nodding, I said, "You know what I think we should do?"

"What?"

"Get some marijuana. How many people have recommended it for my nausea?"

"Everybody. But I thought you were worried about interference with the immunotherapy drugs."

"I was, but I'm less worried now that the combo treatment is done. Besides, I've run out of options."

"I guess we'd better find a doctor to prescribe it then."

Medical marijuana, or medical cannabis, is legal in California, which made me wonder why more doctors' names did not pop up when I did a search. There were only two listed in the Santa Barbara area. One of them saw patients only Tuesday through Thursday, and the other was in Orcutt, 60 miles away, Mondays, Wednesdays, and Fridays.

I called the second one, and the staff person answering the phone informed me that Dr. Flowers had open office hours on Saturdays in Santa Barbara. He invited me to drop in, no appointment necessary, between 1 p.m. and 5 p.m. I said I'd be there.

I returned to the question about why more doctors did not prescribe medical marijuana. Perhaps they prescribed it without advertising to the world, but when I had broached the subject with Dr. Onco, he spoke as if he was not opposed to medical marijuana but would never prescribe it himself. You'd think that if anyone prescribed it, it would be oncologists, whose patients undergoing chemotherapy could benefit from it. But I had never heard of any of my doctors writing a prescription for it. Was it treated as just another drug, or was it kept in the shadows?

While I never asked a doctor directly, I believe the answer lay in the conflict between California and federal law. California law states clearly that the use of medical marijuana, following the appropriate protocol, is legal. However, federal law states that the use of both recreational and medical marijuana is *illegal*.

No matter what California law states, it seemed to me that doctors were not likely to violate federal law and risk their reputation and license. There was nothing to gain and everything to lose, especially in light of the fact that their patients could get medical marijuana from other doctors.

In any event, I planned to see Dr. Flowers on Saturday. Elvira was going to an event that I was not up for, a joint birthday party for Simran and her husband, but Michael offered to take me.

Dr. Flowers had an office in a small house downtown. The door was open to a narrow waiting room with chairs lined up on opposite sides of a coffee table that was almost half the width of the room. Eight people were sitting in the chairs, mostly young and mostly looking quite healthy. There was one middle-aged man sitting alone who wore office attire and looked horribly out of place, as I probably did. I'm not sure what I expected – perhaps the waiting room at the Sansum Clinic Oncology Department – but judging by appearances, I was by far the sickest dude there.

A young man with long hair provided me with a clipboard and the paperwork to fill out. I had also brought documentation of my last two sessions with Dr. Onco. As I filled out the paperwork and Michael was preoccupied with his phone, Dr. Flowers was speaking to patients in his consulting room with the door open. He was talking loudly about different types of marijuana and the various delivery systems, including smoking and edibles. The conversation went on for about ten minutes before the man and woman in the office left with their documentation. They were now authorized to purchase medical marijuana at any dispensary in town.

Our turn came, and the assistant called my name. We entered the office, and Dr. Flowers, who looked to be in his fifties with a moustache and informal manner, rose to shake our hands. He was dressed in khakis and a maroon Nike tee shirt. He instructed me to take the chair beside his desk, and Michael took the chair across from him. As he studied the paperwork I had filled out, I indicated that I was there to quell the nausea from immunotherapy and provided my documentation, but I think it was overkill. He seemed sold on my need from the moment he laid eyes on me.

The conversation centered on the potential benefits of medical marijuana and the delivery method. Dr. Flowers said it was essential to use the whole plant and that the only "proven" delivery method was smoking.

"Or vaping?" Michael asked.

Dr. Flowers nodded, but he was already off on the advantages of juicing and growing one's own plants. He was very knowledgeable, and Michael asked good questions about process, THC versus CBD, and the effects of the different strains. I tried to focus on what technique would help most with the nausea, and Dr. Flowers returned to the purity of smoking the whole plant or vaping the extracted oils.

We were there a long time, much longer than anyone else that morning, but before we left, Dr. Flowers started talking about the latest gaff in the Presidential campaign. He didn't seem to care that the door was open and the words he was using to express his outrage would not normally be uttered in a doctor's office. We smiled and shook his hand as his assistant entered with my personalized authorization to buy medical marijuana.

As we left, we noticed that every chair in the waiting room was taken. The people looked at us as if wondering who had taken up so much time with the doctor, but nobody complained.

We went directly to the dispensary, where they had a staggering array of products. I bought a vape pen on the way home. It looked like a silver pen with a section missing in the middle and a battery at the base. I also bought a cartridge to screw into the missing section and assembled the pieces at home. With Elvira and Michael watching, I activated the vape pen by tapping five times on a button and took a long draw while pushing down on the button. The vapor streamed into my lungs, and I was soon coughing like a kid taking his first hit off a joint. When the laughter died down, we agreed that I should not inhale quite that deeply.

That evening, I took a couple of puffs before dinner, and my stomach, while still fluttering, did not object to Whole Foods Beef Stroganoff. Maybe it was my mind-set as opposed to the marijuana, but whatever the cause, I had a fuller meal than any over the past four days, at least. A little later, because my stomach remained stable, I had a Skinny Cow ice cream sandwich. My taste buds were off, making the ice cream taste like the plastic wrapping it came in, but it was a successful first day with the vape pen.

The next few days were a trial, trying to find the right protocol for the marijuana. First, I didn't like the vaping part, even though it had no aroma. But it caused a burning sensation at the base of my throat and made me cough even with a moderate amount of vapor. I started cautiously, but a few, shallow puffs did not dissipate the nausea. They were also not affecting my brain, either. There was no high or buzzed feeling. I realized that the marijuana had to affect my brain if it was going to help with the nausea.

To get the full benefit, I begin to spend ten to fifteen minutes on the patio, taking somewhere between eight and twelve puffs, depending on whether they were productive or not. Sometimes, I inhaled nothing but air. Most of the time, however, I inhaled vapor and held it in for a few seconds before exhaling. The amount of vapor that came out varied, but I learned that spending that time on the patio was sufficient for the marijuana to make me light-headed and sometimes a little wobbly.

About a half-hour later, I would eat. It was a strange reality because I could eat fairly normally, yet the nausea was still there. It was muffled, like it was hidden under a blanket, but it had not disappeared. I dared not overdo my eating, but I could have a regular meal and not feel as if it was going to come back up through my gullet at any moment.

It was not a perfect situation because I would have loved for the nausea to disappear completely, but it was much better than nothing. With perseverance and a bit of luck, maybe I could even keep up my weight.

TALE OF THE SCALE

On October 13, Sergio sent us a note that they were planning to bring over a treat that evening. The deciding fifth game between the Nationals and Dodgers was on TV. Sergio, Nicole and Eloy arrived in the seventh inning, just in time to watch the Dodgers erupt for four runs. Wearing his Dodger cap, Eloy sat on his papa's lap and was very excited because we were all clapping and yelling encouragements to the TV.

It was scary when the Nationals came back with

two in the bottom of the seventh. Ahead 4-3 in the ninth with runners on first and second, Manager Dave Roberts brought Clayton Kershaw into the game. He got the final two outs in dramatic fashion, and the Dodgers won.

The treat they had brought us was *Caldo de Pollo*, Mexican chicken soup, which made a delicious dinner for two nights. I was able to eat it after vaping. Gayatri had told me that the nausea was in my head, not my body, and it made sense that marijuana helped because it affected my brain. She said she knew many cancer patients, including those she treated, who had benefitted from medical marijuana.

While the medical marijuana didn't work as I thought it might – because the nausea never really disappeared, only slipped into the background – it helped me to eat. At the same time, I didn't want to be stoned all day long.

I tried to get by with the minimum amount of vaping. I would have an eight milligram Zofran pill before breakfast. Zofran had been effective against the nausea when I first started using it, but had stopped working while I was on the combination treatment. It worked again now that I was only on the single drug protocol. About thirty to forty-five minutes before lunch, I would take ten minutes with the vape pen on the patio. There was no odor, no way for anyone to tell if I was inhaling cigarette smoke or medical marijuana, even if there was someone watching. Besides, what I was doing was legal and, if anyone asked, I had documentation to prove it.

I would have another Puff the Magic Dragon session, as Elvira called it, on the patio before dinner. Then I would eat – not as much as when I having five or six meals a day, but hopefully enough to keep up my weight. At 9 p.m., I would take an Ativan, which both settled my stomach and helped me sleep.

As the day approached for my meeting with Dr. Onco, I realized that I displayed many of the characteristics of the complete cancer patient. I was certainly skinny enough, with the pale, sallow look of someone experiencing chemotherapy. My brain was not functioning on all cylinders, and my vision was frequently blurred. Constipation was a regular companion. I had extremely dry, sensitive skin that I couldn't scratch because scratching made it itch more. Dressed in sweats, I lay around the house most of the day, snoozing off and on. My ankles were swollen, so I was now taking Lasix, which made me pee when I wasn't snoozing. And in between the snoozing and the peeing, I was smoking dope so that I could eat chicken soup.

We were nervous on October 19 when we pulled into the Sansum parking lot and went up to Oncology. They always weighed me before going in to see the doctor, and I was worried what the final figure would read this morning.

As usual, after his greetings, Dr. Onco jumped right onto his computer. With an air of disappointment, he revealed my weight: 123 pounds.

"You're at your lowest weight, the same as when we put you on the prednisone."

"I've started using medical marijuana to fight the nausea," I replied. "It's taken me a while to get used to it."

"Is it helping?"

"It is now."

"Was your nausea at its worst right after the treatment last time?"

I hesitated, and Elvira filled the gap.

"Yes, but it got better as time went on."

"Maybe you need more time to recover. For instance, we could set your treatments at every three weeks instead of two."

This idea caused Elvira and me to exchange one of our glances. We knew that Bristol-Myers Squibb recommended a treatment every two weeks.

"If this regimen works," Dr. Onco continued, "we expect you to be on it for a long time. We'll do the CT scans in December to see where we are, but there is no set time for you to come off the Opdivo. That's why it's so important for you to be able to tolerate the side effects. It becomes a quality of life issue"

"How long do you think I'll be on the Opdivo?" I asked.

"We always need to assume the cancer can come back," he said simply. "That's why we don't give an end point."

Dr. Onco turned his attention back to his computer and noted that the results from my cortisol level test had not been received.

"If your adrenal glands are not making enough cortisol, it could be a cause of your nausea. I'll check the results when they come in and let you know if there's a problem."

Elvira and I nodded but did not speak. Dr. Onco stared at his computer pensively.

"I'd like to go ahead with the treatment today," I said.

Dr. Onco paused before saying, "Okay, but I'm putting you on probation."

"Probation?"

"By the next time you come in, which would be – let's see, November 2 – you cannot have lost any more weight. If you have, we'll need to modify your schedule."

Dr. Onco rose, but instead of shaking my hand, he pulled me into a brief hug.

PROBATION

It was time for another trip to Cambria. We needed to get out of the house, and a drive up the coast almost always lifted our spirits.

We turned on our travel music, which was

Everything but the Girl mixed in with k.d. Lang and a group of violinists we had seen perform across the street from the Louvre. The music began to play as we pulled onto Highway 101, heading north according to the signs and west according to the map, an idiosyncrasy of the Santa Barbara area.

I was driving. Over the past three months, Elvira had done almost all our driving, but I had offered to take the wheel for the first part of this trip. It felt good to be in the driver's seat, slicing through the brown, dusty hills under a partly cloudy sky. The sun turned the water various shades of blue. As we neared Gaviota, we could see the cliffs of Hollister Ranch, a beautiful but private spot that surfers loved. It felt as if we were driving right into the ranch until the 101 forced us into an almost 90-degree turn up the slope to the Santa Ynez Valley.

With the coastal view gone, my thoughts wandered, settling on Dr. Onco's comment at our last meeting that I would be taking the Opdivo indefinitely. Did he really mean there was no end point for the Opdivo treatments? And if I would be taking these drugs for the rest of my life, would I also have the side effects?

When I had such thoughts, I remembered what a number of people had said to me, especially my friend Roger: "It's better than the alternative." It had been six months since I started feeling sick, and I realized that people with metastatic melanoma were often dead by this time. With many cancers, especially those in Stage 4, there was a low probability of surviving for six months.

So far, both the immunotherapy treatments and the radiation seemed to be working. I had been able to eat, thanks to the prednisone, and now the medical marijuana was helping muffle the nausea. It was hard to measure the effectiveness of acupuncture, but I believed it benefitted my organs as well as my system as a whole and that it played a role in every step of my progress.

I drove past the turnoff for Highway 1 and up a big hill toward Nojoqui Falls, where Elvira, the boys, and I had hiked many times. We would pass the off-ramp for Buellton and Solvang and even see a corner of the small golf course where we had played 10 or 12 times.

The scenery was predictable; my disease was not. Dr. Onco had given me a road map for projected treatment, but to some extent he was operating on trial and error. The immunotherapy drugs may have extended my life, but their side effects could undermine the process. Also, we didn't know if the break in treatment had slowed my progress. Ideally, my immune system would have carried on the fight against the melanoma on its own, but had it done so? It was impossible to tell.

Maybe this was why I normally didn't spend much time trying to figure out anything but short-term actions and short-term effects. There were too many variables. We just needed to follow the doctor's instructions – after asking numerous penetrating questions – and see what happened. For now, I needed to keep my weight up and get my Opdivo treatment every other Wednesday. By the end of the year, Dr. Onco would order a CT scan to check my body and an MRI to check my brain.

We would just need to hurry up and wait.

The sky remained partly cloudy, and the temperature remained in the low sixties as we made our way north through the Santa Ynez Valley. Vineyards covered most of the land, and we drove through rolling hills covered with vibrant green grape vines. As we approached Santa Maria, Elvira and I joined Tracey Thorn and Ben Watt in singing Tom Waits' "Downtown Train," substituting our own words for the refrain.

The traffic increased through Santa Maria but loosened up again on the other side. On our trips north we would often stop at the Pismo Outlets, but not this day. We confirmed our plans to continue to the Los Osos Valley Road turnoff and stop at the huge shopping center that featured a Home Goods. Not only did it have kitchen mats and bathroom items that we liked, but it had a clean bathroom.

At the shopping center, Elvira went into Old Navy while I stayed outside with my vape pen. I found a semi-private bench around the corner and took some puffs in preparation for lunch in Cambria, about 45 minutes away. I joined Elvira in Home Goods, where she had already found a new kitchen mat and a couple of hand soaps. After finding a dog toy with a working squeaker for Gitana's Christmas gift, we got back on the road – with Elvira driving, of course.

Coming out of the shopping center, we continued west on Los Osos Valley Road, which went from a six-lane to a two-lane road. We turned right on South Bay Boulevard and drove by Montaña de Oro State Park and the Elfin Forest. We connected with Highway 1 in Morro Bay. The sun was high in the sky and shining brightly as the waves curled into shore. Couples were walking along the beach, some with dogs that ran loose on the wide and long beach. On the other side of Morro Bay, the road narrowed to two lanes and proceeded north with a spectacular view of the city and imposing Morro Rock.

It was another 12 miles to Cambria. We arrived at 1:30 p.m., ready for lunch, and went straight to the Main Street Grill.

The big screen sports TV shows in the restaurant led us to yet another discussion of the Dodgers, whose season had finally come to an end. They won two of the first three games against the Cubs in the National League Championship Series, but lost their momentum. In Game 4, the Cubs slaughtered them, 10-2, tying the series at two games apiece. Game 5 was not much better as the Cubs won 8-4. The Cubs needed just one more win, and they got it in Game 6 as the Dodgers were shut out and Clayton Kershaw allowed five runs. It was a disappointing end to the season. Along with every other baseball fan in Los Angeles, we were trying to figure out what had gone wrong and what the Dodgers could do to fix it.

Our order was called, and I retrieved our food. The tri-tip sandwich was thick and meaty, cut in half to make it easy for us to share, and the basket of fries was large. We were both hungry and dove right in. The thinly cut fries were seasoned perfectly, but the tri-tip tasted funny. It was tender with just the right amount of barbecue sauce, but my taste buds were not detecting the usual flavor and my stomach balked at the red meat coming down the chute.

The sandwich tasted good to Elvira, so it was not tainted in any way. Maybe the layers of seared flesh were just too heavy for my digestive system. Another possibility was that I had been overly tentative in my vaping outside Old Navy, and it had not provided its usual buffer against the nausea. Elvira brought up the possibility that my body wasn't used to long car rides, and I might be experiencing motion sickness from the 135-mile trip up the coast.

Whatever the reason, the sandwich was not its usual treat, though I managed to eat almost all of it and shared equally in the consumption of the fries. After eating, we took a short walk downtown before returning to the car and driving across Highway 1 to Moonstone Beach, where we found a spot in the shade to park. With the windows down and an unobstructed view of the ocean, Elvira read while I took a nap.

I felt a little better after resting, but my stomach remained unsettled as we drove to Fiscalini Ranch and our favorite walk. From this boardwalk, we had seen the skies filled with pelicans flying in formation, flanked by seagulls and cormorants. They blotted out the sky and filled the air with screeching, but we never figured out why they had gathered in such numbers. On another occasion, we saw gray and humpback whales migrating north to colder Arctic water, passing so close to shore that we could easily see their tails and bodies without binoculars. Dolphins and otters were also a regular feature on this section of coast, feeding in the kelp beds or swimming gracefully through the breaking waves.

Our ocean view was not as exciting on this day, but I did not complain. It was exciting just to be here. Hell, it was exciting just to be alive.

We walked for about a half-mile and sat on a carved wood bench, which was more picturesque than comfortable. Elvira alertly spotted two spouts in the deep water near the horizon, and otters splashed around in the shallow water near the well-named Otter Cove. After fifteen or twenty minutes, we walked slowly back to the car for the two-and-a-half hour drive to Santa Barbara.

The trip to Cambria tired me out, but I felt okay the next day. My stomach settled down with my usual routine of anti-nausea medicine and vaping, and I continued my efforts to put on weight in anticipation of my November 2 probation meeting with Dr. Onco.

I hadn't weighed myself going into this meeting, so Elvira and I could only guess whether I had met the terms of my probation. My meals had been regular and I'd managed to eat even when I didn't like the taste of the food, but I didn't know if I had done enough to earn my third treatment of Opdivo.

After greeting us amiably, Dr. Onco sat down at

his computer and looked first thing at my weight.

"One hundred twenty-eight pounds," he said. Checking it against last time, he added, "A gain of five pounds."

He did not comment on this information and continued reciting the results of my blood test. He went through every one of the readings, saying "That's good" or "A little high but nothing to worry about". With respect to the test measuring ACTH, which regulates the steroid hormone cortisol, he said that the level was acceptable but they would need to monitor it.

"It could be a cause of your nausea," he explained. He continued to stare at the computer, assimilating the information, and added, "I think I'll recommend the same level of Opdivo as last time."

"I passed probation?" I asked.

"Provisionally," Dr. Onco replied. "I'm still concerned about the nausea."

"I can eat now, thanks to the Zofran and the medical marijuana."

"That's good. But I'm thinking about your quality of life. We don't want you to struggle like you have been. We need to be thinking about how to manage your treatment in the long term."

He paused and looked from Elvira to me.

"We can address that again after we do the tests."

With an encouraging smile, he handed us off to the treatment nurse, Nona, who set up my one-hour packet of Opdivo with a saline flush.

NOVEMBER ARRIVES

Over the next two weeks, which included perhaps the most shocking election in American history, I initiated changes to my routine. The medical marijuana was helping, but I did not enjoy vaping. It was too much like smoking and left me feeling heavy and lethargic. The same was true of the edibles, brownies and gummies, which make me feel like I had a Stonehenge boulder on my back.

Also, the marijuana in any form turned my mind to mush. When we watched *Jeopardy* on TV, Elvira provided ten correct questions to my one.

I gave up on the edibles but began to wonder if I still needed to vape. I was eating much better. Also, Gayatri had said the nausea was in my brain, not my stomach, which was why the marijuana had an effect. If that was so, maybe it was possible to exert the same control on my brain without the marijuana?

I decided to try it. One day, I did not vape. Instead, I took anti-nausea pills before every meal. The experience was different because my brain was not affected, but the nausea did not prevent me from eating. My stomach was fluttering, but was it more unsettled than usual? I wasn't sure.

The next day, I took a Zofran in the morning as

usual and, instead of vaping, took a Reglan before lunch. A few hours later, we took a walk at Hendry's Beach. We had walked several days in a row, but this was the longest and the first on the beach. It was 4 p.m., and the temperature was above 80 degrees. Elvira and I walked two miles, and despite my fluttering stomach, it was wonderful to be on the beach.

These walks had a huge emotional effect on both of us. They were more than a good stretch of the legs; they were an awakening for our bodies and minds, which had stagnated over the course of months. Our last walk in Cambria had been an indicator that I was stronger because I could enjoy the surroundings without getting overly fatigued or sick to my stomach. Walking on the Fiscalini boardwalk was as inspirational as it had ever been.

This inspiration continued when we returned to Santa Barbara. One late afternoon, instead of taking a nap, we decided to take a walk at Shoreline Park. The raised park overlooks the Santa Barbara harbor and has magnificent views of Santa Cruz and Santa Rosa Islands. Exercise had been a regular part of our lives since we met, but neither of us had done much for months. At the park, we walked from the upper parking lot to the area we called the "nub", where we could see surfers catching the early fall waves with the distinctive Santa Barbara wharf and breakwater in the distance.

There was a cool breeze that felt good against our faces. The walk was like liberation from the restrictions on our lives over the past few months, a sense that we were part of a world beyond doctor's offices and treatment centers. Even with all the work that still lay ahead of us, walking on Shoreline Park with the setting sun over the ocean was freedom to us, a moment that was ours and no one else's, a suggestion of life as we had known it and could know it again.

We decided to walk every afternoon at Shoreline Park. The first few days, we did one loop, which was more than a mile; we soon moved on to two loops, which was about 2½ miles. It became an important part of our day, mentally and physically.

At home, of course, I was still trying to figure out my eating regimen. Before dinner, I took a few puffs to settle my stomach before attacking a bison burger with coleslaw. Because sleeping had been difficult the past few nights, I took more puffs before going to bed. It may have helped, but I was still awake for an hour or two in the middle of the night.

The experiment continued on Friday. I had no Zofran in the morning, and it didn't seem to matter as I ate my waffle for breakfast. I did take the Zofran at 11:30 a.m., an hour before lunch. After my acupuncture visit with Gayatri, we went to lunch at Le Café Stella, which offered a delicious lamb sandwich that I hadn't tasted in six months. We both ordered the sandwich with their delicious fries, and it all went down smoothly for me. My sense of taste was still out of whack, but I could taste enough to remember how good the lamb sandwich was.

I continued to test the stability of my stomach at

different meals without taking either the anti-nausea pills or the medical marijuana, but the nausea was unpredictable. One day I'd wake up feeling pretty good and be okay with taking nothing before my meals; the next day, I'd feel funky from the moment I opened my eyes and need a Zofran at lunch and either a Reglan or some puffs before dinner. Many days were a combination. I could handle lunch without the pills or the puffs but not dinner, or vice versa.

Apparently, I was not going to establish a routine. This realization irked me because I liked routines; they helped me feel as if I had control. But this disease and its side effects did not want me to be in control, not even a little bit.

I could live with that. At least, I hoped so.

PART SIX: SCANNING THE HORIZON

THANKSGIVING

As with every year, we counted our blessings as Thanksgiving approached. Immunotherapy was a big one, as was Elvira's constant companionship and support and the support of Michael and Brian, the rest of the family, and our friends. The fact that I could eat a full plate of turkey, mashed potatoes, dressing, gravy, green beans, and salad with family and friends was reason to celebrate.

Kim and Gilbert hosted the affair at their condo clubhouse at the base of Highway 154, a serpentine two-lane road leading through the San Marcos Pass. The Pass meanders past the nearly dry Cachuma Lake to the Santa Ynez Valley, an upscale farming community featuring mini-horses and wineries. It is also home to the Chumash Casino, a favorite gambling spot for everyone from Los Angeles to San Luis Obispo.

The casino had recently undergone a major renovation and now offered overnight accommodations and an elegant restaurant. Neither Elvira nor I had ever been there, except to drive by on our excursions through the Valley. We had been wine-tasting once or twice and olive oil tasting once, always with out-of-town visitors. Los Olivos also offered craft fairs and art-oriented events that we occasionally attended. Afterward, we would usually walk down to J. Woeste, a nursery where Elvira had bought several of her pigs, and eat lunch at the Los Olivos Café. Once we even did a bike ride to Figueroa Mountain, but mostly our trips to the Santa Ynez Valley were for the pleasant drive through the picturesque landscape that we now realized bore a striking resemblance to Tuscany.

Elvira's sister, Sally, had come in from Las Vegas for the holiday, so we picked up her and Aurora late in the afternoon on Thanksgiving Day. I was happy to be driving. Before exiting Highway 154 at Foothill Road, I asked Aurora if she would like to continue up the pass to the Chumash Casino. Her hearing was sketchy at best, and she nodded amiably. When we turned left onto Kim and Gilbert's street, Gilbert was standing in the street directing traffic to the rear of the complex. They had saved us a spot near the entrance to the clubhouse so that Aurora would not need to walk far. As it turned out, she was perfectly comfortable using her wheelchair, which we had brought over her protests, and it was easy to wheel her into the bright room with its upbeat holiday décor.

The Thanksgiving celebration, which we had

hosted at our house many times when we lived in Goleta, was an amalgam of family, extended family, former family, girlfriends, boyfriends, and friends of the family. Generally, I would know about three-quarters of the attendees but would have a conversation with only about half. I felt conspicuous this time because of my appearance. I was still down almost 20 pounds and a little weak, and my clothes sagged like they were on a hanger. Plus, my eyebrows and eyelids had changed color; Elvira maintained my new color was "wheat" while it looked like creeping white hair to me. Either way, those who hadn't seen me in a long time or didn't know I was sick would probably think I looked weird.

No one seemed to care. Kim had a bad cold but hugged us all with face averted and scurried around to ensure everything was in place. While Dr. Onco had told me that my immune system was so pumped up that it would probably be hard for bacteria or a virus to penetrate it, I was careful about being too much in the presence of sick people. After all, the same Dr. Onco had told me I didn't need a flu shot but that Elvira should probably get one, whether for her own health or mine, we didn't know. Also, the one time I'd landed in the hospital, my diagnosis was gastroenteritis, or the flu, and that was after I'd started the combination immunotherapy treatment.

Geronimo was excited to see me after the long lay-off. When Gilbert had finished directing traffic, he came in and threw his arms around me. He wanted to hear how the recovery was going and also to talk about the emotional trauma of cancer among his friends. Our conversation was cut short by the

153

announcement of dinner. Elvira and I sat at a table with Michael, Brian, Tina, and Rachel. Others came and went in the remaining seats. Aurora sat at the head of the biggest table, the matriarch of the family, and was served her favorite Thanksgiving foods along with a glass or two of wine.

Rumor was that it had been prepared by a local health food restaurant that had a reputation for organic products and high prices. The food was laid out in chaffing dishes on draped 3' x 6' tables. Even with my limited ability to smell, the aroma of turkey, mashed potatoes, stuffing, and gravy hit me full force. There was also cranberry sauce, green beans, and green salad.

It was a delicious meal, and it was important for me simply to feel normal again. It had been a long time since I was able to hobnob with a large group of people while eating a full meal with seconds and dessert. The conversation was only peripherally about my health because, I believe, people could see that I was functional. I was thin but not so thin that someone would think they should be ready to call 911 at any moment. I was also eating a plate as full as theirs. Much of the table conversation was carried by Mike, a family member by remarriage, who had endured his share of health problems and was due for hip surgery in a few days. Instead of talking about his hip, however, he told stories about mountain climbing and boat trips that were diverting and interesting, evoking similar tales from others around the table.

On holiday get-togethers, it was Aurora's call when to leave, but I grew tired as the afternoon turned into evening. I asked her if she was ready, and she looked at me eagerly as if to say, "It's about time someone suggested it." As Elvira and I were thanking our hosts, others ushered Aurora to the car.

We were tired when we arrived home, especially me. We had recorded the National Dog Show from the Kennel Club in Philadelphia and sat listlessly in front of the TV to watch it. We were rooting for the corgi, which made the finals, but the greyhound, also a beautiful dog, took home best in show. Amazingly, we were still awake at the end.

BLACK FRIDAY AND RAINY SATURDAY

Elvira had now been retired almost four years and me for three-and-a-half. As a result, long weekends didn't have the significance they did when we needed to trudge back to work on the following Monday. Thanksgiving weekend, however, still had a special feel to it with its emphasis on family and food, both of which had a special place in our hearts.

We did not go shopping on Black Friday. We had done most of our Christmas shopping already on a trip to Camarillo and going online. Also, Elvira was planning to make her seasoned pretzels to give away.

Three years earlier, we had gone shopping after eating Thanksgiving dinner. It was the holiday season before we left on our Europe trip, and we needed luggage. We found a great deal at Macy's, even as we felt sorry for the sales associate for having to work on the holiday.

I woke up on Friday with a food hangover, or maybe just lingering fatigue from the activity of the day before. I stayed in bed most of the morning even though I could see that it was a beautiful day outside, sunny in the upper 60s. Elvira was moving slowly as well, sipping coffee and feeling pleasantly entertained by her iPad. I had cereal with blueberries, banana, and almond milk followed by a piece of toast and small cup of coffee. The coffee had been a breakthrough because I never thought it would taste good to me again. I realized that the reason I could drink it might be that my sense of smell and taste was suppressed, but that was okay. Having coffee in the morning was another welcome return to the normalcy of life.

After breakfast, I hooked up the laptop and tried to shake off my lethargy by working on my journal. I had made it to Part Four. It was a challenge to find the right language. It was the time when the combination treatments of immunotherapy seemed to be working and the melanoma seemed to be retreating, but my body was falling apart. I was losing weight and growing weaker. That period was depressing and uplifting at the same time, and describing those complex feelings was difficult.

I kept rewriting the same passages, trying to come up with the right words, and finally gave up. Maybe it was my sluggishness that was keeping me from making progress. I would try again on Saturday, when this washed-out feeling would hopefully be gone and I would have more energy.

It was already lunchtime, and I had my usual

turkey tacos. I varied my lunch menu when we had leftovers from dinner the night before, but turkey tacos were the mainstay of my post-prednisone diet. I never seemed to tire of them.

We did little the remainder of the day and had a simple dinner. The rest day seemed to help because I felt better on Saturday. After breakfast, I sat down at my laptop and made it through the passage that had given me so much trouble the day before. It happened that way sometimes with writing. What seemed impossible one day became manageable the next. This was not to say that I found the perfect language, only that I was comfortable with how I had conveyed my feelings during that difficult time. I would not know if it made sense until Elvira read it and made her suggestions.

Lunch tasted better after the successful session at my laptop. While I still had no set routine for my anti-nausea measures, I had eliminated vaping during the day. If my stomach felt queasy before lunch, I would take a Zofran; if my stomach felt queasy before dinner, I would take a Reglan. Some days, I took both; some days, I took neither. I was eating full meals now and continued to put on weight, though the gains were slow. At least, I was solidly in the 130s. I would only vape in the evening if the itchiness, the other side effect that had stayed with me from the combination immunotherapy days, would not let me sleep. Then I would slip into the bathroom and take five to seven puffs, which would usually allow me to ignore the itchiness and fall asleep.

As it rained steadily on Saturday, we watched football and enjoyed the pitter-patter on our roof. Elvira would get occasional tweets from the boys. Brian had taken a boat trip to Santa Cruz Island, where he dived for a variety of fish. He returned just as the rain was beginning. Michael was visiting his good friend, Klark, at Mammoth and snowboarding down slopes that he would only tell his mother about when he was safely at the bottom. While Elvira and I looked forward to taking our own trips someday, we were glad that our sons were having their own outdoor adventures.

Rain was a special treat in Santa Barbara, now in its fifth year of drought. It seemed as if getting just a few inches a year, even as the rest of the country seemed to be awash in rain, was becoming the norm. Elvira placed our plants in perfect position to get maximum watering, and we had taken our Honda SUV out of the carport so it could get washed. The rain lasted most of the day and through dinner as Elvira crushed me on *Jeopardy* questions again. (I couldn't blame the medical marijuana this time.) Afterward, Elvira watched TV in the living room, and I watched two of my favorite classic movies in the bedroom: *Tootsie* and *El Dorado*.

All in all, it had been a slow day, conducive to having one's mind wander. Mine wandered directly to the question that would drive me crazy if I asked it every day: Was I still getting better? Since my last scan, when improvement was discernible throughout my body, I had been taken off treatment for six weeks, gone through a prednisone regimen, and gone onto a single immunotherapy drug instead of the combination treatment. Dr. Onco was confident that my body was still waging an assault on the cancer cells, but these drugs were so new and the treatment so unpredictable that it was impossible to know for sure what was happening.

The signs remained positive. I felt better, could eat more, and had no apparent recurrence of the epidermal tumors on my back or lymph node. These factors eased my doubts and helped me share Dr. Onco's confidence about my upcoming CT scan and MRI, which he would schedule at our next meeting.

RESTORING CHRISTMAS

Uncle Frank came in on Sunday, but his dog Gitana was not herself from the beginning of the visit. She was limping and scratching continuously. She still wanted to go for a walk, of course, and I took her through the swale behind our house up to the More Mesa bluffs. She walked at half-speed, stopped to scratch repeatedly, and seemed only mildly interested in other dogs and people. When we returned, I described her behavior, and Frank said it had been like that lately. He was concerned because of the history of dysplasia for Aussies and Aussie mixes of Gitana's age. He had already had both her hips surgically repaired, but he knew too well from previous experience that there was a limit to surgery's ability to remedy the problem.

Gitana's health issues cast a shadow over Frank's usually upbeat visit, but he called the next day to explain at least part of her behavior – she had fleas. For years, Frank had been zealous in his preventive actions against fleas, but he had finally relaxed. He was convinced she would never get them. Unfortunately, she had managed to defy the odds of her having her first infestation at the age of ten and had come down with a doozy. Frank took her to the vet for a bath and washed down the parts of the house where she lay, especially her beds. He was flabbergasted but also in a way pleased because at least there was an explanation for the incessant scratching. When she was finally rid of the fleas, her limp seemed less severe and she seemed like a happier dog in general.

On Monday, I did my bloodwork in preparation for Wednesday's meeting with Dr. Onco. Later that day, Elvira went to see Gayatri, who had offered to treat her without payment. Having treated Elvira long before she treated me, Gayatri wanted to help her and knew we couldn't afford acupuncture for both of us. The money didn't matter to her, but our health did. Elvira went for a session and was scheduled for one every month afterward.

Although I have mentioned that our Christmas shopping was done, we each had one item left to buy. We had decided that in addition to the set of moderately priced items we normally purchased, we would give each other something we would never buy for ourselves. Elvira decided that she wanted an upscale Dodger jacket that I could get online. After reflection, I asked for a desk or at least a table on which I could set my laptop. I had been moving the laptop from spot to spot in the house, and that was fine, but I had been on it a lot lately and missed having one spot to place the laptop along with my printer, paper, and other materials.

At first, Elvira thought a desk was not fun, but I tried to convince her that having a comfortable spot for my writing was perfect for me. It would not only help me be more productive, it would be an affirmation, a statement that we believed I would keep writing long after this journal was finished. I had novels to produce, and I would need a place to do that next year and the year after that, and so on. A desk was a gift that spoke to my future as a writer as well as our future together, and that was what I wanted.

Elvira's jacket had a similar meaning. She intended to wear it to all the future Dodger games we would go to in the upcoming years.

We set Tuesday, while our house was being cleaned, as the day to search for an appropriate desk or table. We went to several stores that sold desks, but they were cheap-looking and way overpriced. We went to the only used furniture store we knew in the area, and the items there were also overpriced. I wanted something simple and functional and didn't want Elvira to pay a lot of money. We were having no luck, even with a table that would serve the purpose.

On our way back from the big box stores in Goleta, we decided to stop at the Habitat for Humanity ReStore. The manager explained that they usually did not stock desks, but he had a few that might work for home use. He led us to a slightly used and darkly stained hardwood Steelcase desk. The drawers rolled in and out as if they had been oiled the day before, and the minor scratches on the surface could easily be covered by my accessories. When he quoted the price, it was within our range. We put a hold on it and kept looking for about an hour before deciding. We would take it, as long as we could fit it into our house.

Surprisingly, the desk fit into the back of our CR-V, and I tipped the four ReStore movers who loaned us their four-wheel dolly. We asked them if they'd come home with us to unload it, but that was going too far. Then we drove home at about 20 miles per hour. We backed in so that we could unload on the driveway by the path leading to our front door. With a full set of drawers on both sides, the desk was not only heavy, it was cumbersome. We managed to slide it from the CR-V onto the dolly, but moving it across the asphalt driveway even for a few feet was not easy. Every seam and crack in the concrete path stopped the wheels while the desk's momentum almost threw if off the dolly. We finally made it to the front door, where we tried to move the desk onto its side. It slid off the dolly, crushed a cactus, and concussed a metal goose in our small yard before we could right it again.

"Do you need some help?" Mary called from next door.

We admitted that we did.

She called her husband John, an engineer, and the two of them helped us not only get the desk onto the dolly on its side, but over the threshold and into our living room. It was clear that the desk would not fit in the study, so we decided to put it in the sun room. We tried several rearrangements of the furniture before placing it in front of the picture window. We had to replace our rustic 3' by 6' coffee table with a round one 17" in diameter, but the desk fit perfectly with that minor adjustment.

It was a wonderful Christmas gift. Not wrappable, of course, but we put a bow on it. I stuffed the drawers with my paraphernalia and used my laptop on it later that day. It was more than I ever could have wished for, and Elvira was pleased at the new look of our sun room.

DR. ONCO SETS THE DATE

On the day of our meeting with Dr. Onco, I awoke at 4 a.m., itching like a madman. I had given in to an itch here and there, and soon I was scratching all over my body, making it itch even more. The itchiness was a side effect of the Opdivo and associated with my body getting hot. The heat could come from the outside, like a hot shower or our fireplace, or the inside, like from sugar-laden food. Stress might have had something to do with it as well.

I scratched my arms, thighs, ankles, chest, back, and scalp. It felt blissful while I was doing it, like a dog scratching in just the right spot, but the itchiness returned with fervor as soon as I stopped. I finally got up around 4:30 because it was impossible to sleep while riding this merry-go-round. I slathered my body with the lotion Dr. Dermo had prescribed and ate an early breakfast as the itchiness gradually moved to the back of my consciousness.

By the time we left for Sansum, I had recovered from my spell and was focused on this last meeting before the CT scan and MRI. Dr. Onco greeted us and proceeded to relate that my weight was up three pounds and vital signs were all good except for the pituitary gland output. It had been marginal before but now was below normal. He explained that the pituitary gland, which is only the size of a pea, secretes hormones that help control growth, blood pressure, the thyroid gland's activities, the metabolism, and more. It was like the captain of the glands, and if it wasn't producing its hormones, the body did not function normally.

"We'll need to keep an eye on that," Dr. Onco said, apparently not worried about any immediate consequences. "Now, let's see about scheduling your tests."

He set up my CT scan and MRI back-to-back on December 13, the day before my next meeting with him. He typed the information into the computer.

"All set up," he said with satisfaction. "We'll go ahead with your treatment today. The nurse will come get you from the waiting room."

He smiled and shook our hands, and we returned to the waiting room, which was more crowded than usual. In fact, we could not find seats and waited by the door, which was where we encountered Bud, my partner in a treatment room several weeks earlier. He was in a wheelchair and seemed tired and weak. We talked for a minute before his name was called. His wife mentioned that he was getting the same combination Yervoy-Opdivo regimen that I'd had. We said encouraging things, but we were worried.

We waited a long time before getting into a treatment room and, once there, had to wait for a pump to become available. The RNs were rushing around attending to their patients, and it was a new nurse, Katie, who finally managed to bring in a pump and set up my Opdivo treatment. The session took an hour, with another ten minutes for the saline flush, but the total time we had been there was more than three hours. I think Elvira was happy to hear that I was hungry afterward because she had grown hungry herself waiting in that small room for the drip-drip-drip to finally end. We had a special deal at a Chinese restaurant in Five Points, where we split two dishes along with fried rice.

I was sluggish the rest of that day and the next, but it was nothing compared to my lethargy following the combination treatments. There also seemed to be less sluggishness following every subsequent Opdivo treatment.

On Thursday evening, we celebrated Brian's thirty-second birthday at Aurora's house. We had Mexican food and a long discussion about the nature of generations. Brian maintained that generations could be measured from the Baby Boomers at twenty-year intervals. In his view, the Baby Boomers were those born between 1945 and 1964, Generation X was born between 1965 and 1984, and Millennials were born between 1985 and 2004. By this metric, Brian, who was born in 1984, considered himself part of Generation X.

Elvira pointed out that he had a lot more in common with the Millennials than with the Gen Xers, everything from his world view to his computer expertise. He disagreed, and the discussion continued as Rachel and I threw in occasional comments. Aurora listened comfortably from her armchair, dropping off every so often as the evening grew later. Rachel, Elvira and I left around 9 p.m., and Brian stayed, it being his night to stay with his grandma.

On Friday, I had my session with Gayatri, and Elvira and I stopped at Whole Foods on the way home. She chose cod from one of their prepared food counters, and I bought two slices of pepperoni pizza, which I ate as we watched Tiger Woods's return from obscurity. We had watched him play frequently during his amazing run of wins and were eager to see what was left of the phenomenal player he had been. There were flashes of the old brilliance, but in the end he faded as younger players who had not endured three back surgeries claimed the leaderboard. Even with his liabilities, however, he was fun to watch.

AN INDEFINITE ARTICLE

We woke up on Saturday before 8 a.m., and later

that morning Elvira made French toast from challah bread with turkey sausage on the side. We ate while watching golf and reading the news on our iPads. On this morning, I was struck by an article in *The New York Times* entitled "Immune System, Unleashed by Cancer Therapies, Can Attack Organs" by Matt Richtel.

The first example in the article described the severe reaction to combination immunotherapy of a sixty-one-year-old man with melanoma. This example illustrated the risks associated with drugs that activated the immune system to attack cancer cells. He noted that the bowels, liver, lungs, kidneys, pancreas, and adrenal and pituitary glands were all potential victims of immunotherapy drugs. Diabetes could be another effect of this regimen.

The author went on to detail how dangerous the treatment could be even as it was saving lives. He provided numerous examples of people who had suffered serious side effects. He stated – in my words – that doctors needed to remain aware of the side effects and weigh the benefit of the new drugs against the potential organ failure and diabetes. His point was well-taken, but I believed most patients were like me. I was given full warning of the possible side effects, from minor to catastrophic, and still there was no doubt in my mind, not to mention Elvira's, that we wanted the drugs. I would almost certainly be dead by the end of 2016 without Yervoy and Opdivo and the management of these drugs by Dr. Onco.

Mr. Richtel's article counter-balanced a lot of the news, including numerous articles in *The New York*

Times, about immunotherapy's miraculous effects. It was a good reminder that these drugs were medicine, not a miracle cure. On the other hand, it was important to remember all the good the drugs were doing. The fact that they could cause my pituitary gland to fail or give me diabetes or even a heart attack was a reason for me and my doctors to be watchful and careful, not to turn our backs on the most promising cancer treatment in recent history.

I shared the article with Roger and Sheryl, who came up from Riverside the next day for a visit. As we walked at Shoreline Park, Roger, the biologist, shrugged and agreed with me that it was important to be aware of side effects but even more important not to lose track of the primary objective, which was to combat the cancer. He added that new medicines were never perfect, and doctors and researchers were still learning about them even as they were being used by the general population. It was a natural process and one that would likely be repeated as the immunotherapy method was applied to the treatment of other cancers.

It was approaching sunset when we finished our walk and stopped at the top end of the park. We watched the sun turn liquid, melting into the horizon as the clouds turned a brilliant peach color and the blue of the ocean changed from shiny to matte. We all got out our iPhones, and the three of them took pictures of the sunset while I took a picture of them taking a picture of the sunset.

We had dinner at Lure, the newest – and some say the best – fish restaurant in town. Elvira had the seabass, Sheryl and I had the trout almandine, and Roger had the fish sampler. It was my first dinner at a cloth-napkin restaurant in months. We made it back-to-back meals the next morning by having a full breakfast at Esau's in Carpinteria. We visited Gallup and Stribling nursery afterward, where the colorful diversity and the sheer number of the orchids were almost overwhelming.

Roger and Sheryl left from there for Riverside, and we went home. I was tired but pleased not only to see our friends, but that I had been able to eat so robustly. At home, we watched the end of the golf tournament, and I read. I had avoided reading books while I was sick, and Elvira recommended two for me. The first one I read was a light detective novel by Andrea Camilleri entitled *A Voice in the Night*, set in Sicily. The second was an even lighter but clever detective novel by Spencer Quinn entitled *Scents and Sensibility*. This was the seventh novel in Quinn's series, where the stories were told from Chet's point of view. Chet was the detective's dog.

MORE FRIENDS AND TRAVELS WITH CHARLEY

Tuesday marked Day 7 on the countdown to the CT scan and MRI and Day 8 until we met with Dr. Onco. Elvira and I were both starting to get nervous, as we had in September. This set of tests would reveal whether or not my immune system had continued to attack the cancer cells after the cessation of the combination therapy. It would also reveal whether or not the Opdivo was holding its own against the melanoma.

We filled up our days as best we could. On Tuesday, we had lunch with Ann and Jon. Ann was a member of the group with whom I was scheduled to have lunch back in July but had a dizzy spell that prevented me from going. She was also my editor and a very good one. Jon was a recently retired professor of economics at UCSB and a golf buddy. We had arranged lunch not only to visit with them but for me to give Ann about 50 pages of this journal for her to edit.

After lunch, we ran errands and ended up at Marie's. She had returned from visiting her sister in Minnesota and immediately made more of her exquisite spaghetti sauce. We caught up on everything from the aftermath of the election to the fact that a Sprouts market had replaced the Von's in Goleta. While I was fine during these outings, I was tired when we got home, my stamina coming back slowly. That evening, we had spaghetti for dinner, watched the newest Jason Bourne movie on pay-per-view, and went to bed.

December 7 was Pearl Harbor Day, and as usual we thought about all the people who lost their lives on that horrendous surprise attack on the American naval base in Hawaii. I also thought about my father, who served in the Army in World War II. He was not a talkative man, but he was especially uncommunicative about his war years. He did reveal at one point that he had a bad experience in Okinawa, perhaps shooting at a civilian who was shooting at the

American soldiers. It was unclear what had happened, and I spoke to my brother Steve. He remembered hearing something similar from Dad, and our conversation evolved into a discussion of his life.

Tom Wieneke had died in 1991. How much the war shaped Dad's personality was impossible to determine. Steve and I remembered him as a good man who was smart and worked hard, but was taciturn and aloof much of the time. He lost his father in a train accident at an early age and was raised by a very stern mother. He had been a Triple-A baseball player, a switch-hitting second baseman whose knees gave out before he could make it to the majors. When my brothers and I were young, we had over-the-line games where Dad and I took on Dave and Steve. Both right-handed and left-handed, Dad would hit spectacular home runs that I remember soaring impossibly into the sky. He also coached us in Little League, and Mom would keep score for us. She would also keep a scrapbook on each of us that extended from our earliest days of playing organized sports.

Steve and I agreed that those were the best memories of our childhood as we did something as a family without rancor or heavy demands. In that setting, we were accepted for who we were, not what we did, and we treasured those moments to this day.

It was interesting that even as we discussed the effect of war on our father, Steve was dealing with his own issues from serving in Vietnam. He had been traveling for two years after retiring from managing water districts, writing about his life following the war and trying to understand how that experience had shaped him as a person. We talked about it at least once a week, as well as the battle that I was waging against a different type of enemy.

That evening, I started a new book that, coincidentally, was set in 1961, the year I began Little League baseball. It was John Steinbeck's *Travels with Charley in Search of America*. I had read it long ago and enjoyed it but didn't remember much about it. Starting at his home in Sag Harbor at the age of 52, driving a camper he named after Rocinante, Don Quixote's horse, and in the company of a French Poodle named Charley, Steinbeck traveled north into the far reaches of Maine, where he struck up conversations with strangers he would otherwise never have known. He was trying to understand the people who work and live in a nation that was undergoing great change. He felt the change but did not understand it, and he hoped to get a handle on it through conversations with people everywhere he went.

From Maine he drove east to Niagara Falls and through portions of Pennsylvania, Ohio, and Indiana. After taking a short break in Chicago, he continued west through Minnesota and North Dakota. He loved the back-to-nature feel of Montana and was shocked at the expansion of Seattle. He headed south to his old haunts in California, where he had grown up and which serves as the setting to several of his most famous novels, including *Cannery Row* and *Tortilla Flat*. From there, he drove east through Texas and finally the South, where he witnessed a disturbing example of segregation.

While three months of traveling in a camper can hardly give one a comprehensive understanding of America, Steinbeck identified numerous trends that we recognize today. Certainly, the transition from rural life to city life has not only continued, but accelerated. He recognized the vanishing regionalism that had formerly characterized the U.S. He could see that everything from speech to the stores where we buy our food was becoming standardized. He was depressed by the standardization of America and saw way too much plastic. He avoided interstate highways and freeways because he didn't want to drive from New York to California without seeing anything.

Despite the increasing standardization throughout the country, Steinbeck did notice the distinct differences between people on the coast and in the middle of the country. He could not possibly have foreseen the great divide reflected in the election of 2016, but he was smart enough to see the beginnings of it.

It was a thoughtful and entertaining read, and I was pleased that I decided to pick it up again after all these years. The book was probably fifteen years old when I first read it, and now it was more than fifty. Amazing.

THE DAY THE EARTH STOOD STILL

Elvira made a delicious chicken pot pie that night, and we ate it with a glass of chardonnay. The wine might not have tasted the same to me as it had before, but it complemented the dinner perfectly.

I was itchy later, however, and decided to take a Benadryl to take the edge off and allow me to sleep better. Bad decision. It seemed to have the opposite effect, making me slightly edgy. It took me a long time to fall asleep; as a result, I slept in till 10 a.m., which was when Elvira went for a walk around our neighborhood with Lynn. I stumbled out of bed, feeling lazy. Elvira and I hung around the house all day, having the rest of the chicken pot pie over smashed potatoes. I was sure it was very good even though I couldn't taste much and my stomach was jittery.

I didn't know what to make of my condition except to ask whether I was getting ahead of myself with recovery expectations. I felt strongly that I was on an upward arc, but maybe I wasn't as far along as I thought. Should I be feeling this funky if the melanoma was on the run and I was taking only one immunotherapy drug? Maybe, maybe not. Dr. Onco probably wouldn't know, either, because whenever I asked him if I *should* be feeling this way or that way, he replied that each patient was different. There was no "should" in this process.

The idea of getting a check-up in six days may also have had an effect. Elvira and I both seemed nervous.

On Friday, we had the pleasant distraction of Eloy coming to visit – with his parents, of course. I had slept better, taking only Ativan an hour before going to bed. After sandwiches, we went down to the small playground in our complex, and Eloy was thrilled with the jungle gym. He wanted Sergio to be on the top level with him, and every time he went down the slide, he wanted one of us to follow him. Nicole, Elvira and I each took our turns, not fitting quite as well as Eloy but getting down successfully to a round of applause.

The next few days were quiet on the outside and tumultuous on the inside. A big social event was on Saturday night: Lois Capps's party celebrating her retirement from Congress after eighteen years. We spent much of the time with Walter's brothers, Roger and Doug, and their wives, Jan and Liz. I also spoke with Reza, who in 1996 had the enthusiasm of fifty volunteers, and Ben, who once raised money by performing as a human juke box. On Sunday, Elvira and I took a leisurely drive out Highway 192 on a clear, crisp afternoon. That evening, we began our Christmas season movie tradition by watching *It's a Wonderful Life*.

I got my bloodwork done on Monday morning and picked up the barium I would need to drink before the CT scan. Elvira stayed busy during the day by making the seasoned pretzels she gave away at Christmas. The term most often applied to the pretzels was "addictive". She also made a delectable pasta dish for dinner using rockfish that Brian had caught near the Channel Islands. As usual, we ate while watching *Jeopardy*, at which I was becoming better, answering two questions to Elvira's ten instead of just one. Later, we watched *The Grinch Who Stole Christmas* (the animated version with Boris Karloff), and I drank one of my pints of barium. It was supposedly vanilla flavored, but whoever labeled it must have had taste buds worse than mine.

Tuesday, December 13, was the day of my tests. I ate nothing and drank my second pint of barium in the morning. Elvira drove us to Sansum. The MRI was first, in an outdoor trailer, presumably so the noise didn't shake the building. It went off without a hitch. The same with the CT scan, during which I lay perfectly still every time I was prompted by the computer-generated voice. When we came home, I had cereal.

It was a very long day. We had a walk in the late afternoon, which allowed us to breathe easier for a while, but our nervousness was almost palpable as our meeting the next morning with Dr. Onco approached.

When we arrived at Sansum, Elvira delivered 24 packets of seasoned pretzels, one for each of the employees of the Oncology/Hematology Department, including the doctors. We were told Dr. Onco had not arrived yet and were ushered into his office to wait.

Each room in the clinic seemed to have a theme, and this one could have been eagles because there were two carved wooden eagles on the corner table. However, there was also a print on the wall of what appeared to be an English garden, painted in pastels. On another wall was a wedding photo, taken from behind, of newlyweds walking hand-in-hand. Elvira and I have a picture like that of us on the beach, but I wondered what eagles, an English garden, and a picture of newlyweds had in common. The explanation could have been that these were photos with which Dr. Onco wanted to adorn his office, but that explanation was too easy. I needed something more complex to ponder until the doctor arrived.

Dr. Onco finally entered the room and shook hands with us, but it was obvious from the beginning that something was on his mind. It did not take long for us to learn what it was.

"I just spoke with the radiologist," he said. "There's a problem with your bladder."

"My bladder?"

"Yes. It needs to be addressed immediately, but let's go over your test results first."

We were stunned. Our hopes for a nothing-but-good-news day evaporated instantly.

As if he had not said anything about my bladder, Dr. Onco sat down at the computer and began the normal meeting ritual. He noted my weight, which was up two pounds to 136, and vital signs, which were all stable. He went through the results of the MRI and scan very quickly. No spots were found on my brain, back, lymph node, lungs, pancreas, colon, or leg. The kidney and liver were not clear, however, and he could not tell how much of the residual spots were dead tissue. The doctor categorized the results not as remission, which Elvira and I had hoped for, but a partial response.

When he was finished, the doctor turned to us with a serious expression. For the first time that day turned the computer screen so that we could see it.

"Here's what I mean about your bladder," he said, manipulating the mouse. "See this shadow? It could be a hemorrhagic clot or a cyst or debris, we're not sure. It could also be neoplasm."

"What's neoplasm?" I asked.

"It's abnormal growth of cells or tissue that could be cancer."

His words hit us like a load of bricks.

"As I say, it could also be a clot or a cyst, but we need to check it out through a urologist."

"Dr. Uro," I muttered.

"Pardon me?"

"Dr. Uro is my urologist."

"We can check with him. He might be taking some time off."

"I've also seen Dr. Peters."

"I'll ask our staff to set it up."

Elvira shook her head slightly as if waking up and asked, "Do you think it's the melanoma?"

"No, I don't," Dr. Onco replied. "It wouldn't make sense for the melanoma to be retreating everywhere else, including the kidney, and advancing in his bladder. If it's cancer, it's localized."

I thought about that for a moment.

"But if the immunotherapy is keeping cancer out of the kidney, shouldn't it also work on the bladder? They're right next to each other."

"We really don't know much about how those drugs interact with new cancers," Dr. Onco admitted. "And that is what it would be in the bladder. We'll need to wait for the urologist's report."

We sat in silence for a moment. It was Dr. Onco who broke it.

"We'll get to the bottom of this as soon as we can. In the meantime, there's no reason you can't have your treatment today."

He turned to his computer screen. I took a deep breath and glanced at Elvira, who smiled ruefully. When Dr. Onco finished typing, he rose from his chair and extended his hand.

We exited and were ushered into the waiting room. After a few minutes, Chris called my name and led us into the treatment room. He inserted the IV on the first try and began the saline drip before exiting to prepare the Opdivo.

When Elvira and I were alone, I said, "In a way, we're back where we started."

"What do you mean?"

"Dr. Uro wanted to do a cystoscopy way back at the beginning of this mess. I didn't want him to do it, remember? I've had two before, and that's enough for a lifetime."

A cystoscopy was the test where a tube was extended through the urethra into the bladder. It was the test that sadistic doctors had used more than fifty years earlier to torture my brother, Dave. At least, they seemed sadistic at the time as I watched my brother suffer over and over again without a diagnosis. The tests and the medicine were physically and mentally traumatic for him and the rest of the family.

This situation was different, of course. There was an anomaly that could be cancer. They had no choice but to go in and I had no choice but to consent. It was also fifty years ago that Dave had his cystoscopies, and they were less traumatic when I had one as a precaution seven or eight earlier. Still, I shuddered not only at the idea of having bladder cancer but at the test to determine whether or not I had it.

"It seems like a lifetime ago that we were talking about your having a cystoscopy," Elvira said. After a pause, she added, "But we are back where we started, and in more than one way."

I knew what she meant, that our lives could be changing again due to cancer. It was odd that the word should have such import with us when we had been living with melanoma for more than six months, but the melanoma seemed to be retreating. This new growth, if it was cancer, was sprouting while I was undergoing treatment and supposedly getting better. Did this mean I would need to start all over again with new treatments? If so, was there a miracle immunotherapy drug for bladder cancer? Probably not.

The load of bricks remained heavy on us as we sat in the treatment room, waiting for Chris to return.

TEST WITH A CAUSE

After my treatment, we checked with the scheduling nurse to see if she'd had any luck with a urologist appointment. To our surprise, she had managed to get an appointment with Dr. Peters for 8:30 the following morning.

"At least we won't need to wait long," Elvira said.

We went home and tried to act normal, each of us pretending not to be scared. We watched *Law & Order* episodes most of the day and stayed up late in the hope we would be tired enough to sleep. We dropped off without a problem, but we were both awake much of the night.

Long before it was time to get up, my eyes popped open and I felt the deep, hollow sinking feeling that I had known so well as a child. It was brought on by the specter of death, but also the fear of loneliness. Elvira had traveled every step of this journey with me, but I could not help but think that this might be the separation point. The thought of being without her was terrifying, the loneliest thought I had ever had, and I could not turn it off till the morning light began to brighten the room.

We arrived early at Dr. Peters' office and sat in the waiting room. Several people were called before us, a surprise because I didn't think they made appointments before 8:30 a.m. I was finally called around 8:45, and I left Elvira with a kiss as she wished me good luck. I followed the assistant through the labyrinth to the procedure room. It was larger than I remembered with a lone table in the center and equipment all around it as if they were planning to build the Frankenstein monster. After the assistant confirmed my ID and explained the procedure, he led me to the table and instructed me to drop my shorts and lie on my back.

When I was situated as instructed, he placed a towel on my private parts so that I could not see. There was a stinging sensation, but it wasn't as awful as I thought it might be and it and didn't last long. When the assistant stood up, he asked, "Are you nervous?"

"A little."

"You should be okay if you didn't have any reaction to what I've already done."

I nodded, wondering what he had done. Then I decided it was best not to wonder – or know. I was trying to think of something else when Dr. Peters entered the room. He was a man in his fifties with a thin face and olive skin. He smiled pleasantly.

"Dr. Onco sent you over to see me," he said.
"The scan found some sort of abnormality with your
bladder."

"Yes."

"Well, let's have a peek then, shall we?"

He walked to the end of the table and began the
procedure. An interesting dimension of the
cystoscopy was that the camera at the end of the
plastic tube being pushed through my urethra
projected onto a monitor that I could see at the same
time as the doctor. It was like when Dr. Onco turned
his computer monitor around so that Elvira and I
could see what he saw as he searched for cancerous
spots, only this time it was a moving picture.

The tube made its way quickly through my
urethra into my bladder. It was like walking through
a maze of alleys to get to an intersection. When he
reached the bladder, the lining looked like bubble
wrap, which didn't seem good to me, but Dr. Peters
was right there with an explanation.

"That's normal," he said without hesitation. He
moved the tube to the right, which felt weird on my
insides but didn't hurt.

"Do you see that area that looks different" he
asked. "Right there."

"Yes."

"That's your prostate. It's encroaching on your bladder. That's what caused the shadow on the scan."

"It is?"

"Yes, it is. The bladder itself looks normal, and there's no sign of cancer. You just have one king-sized prostate."

I smiled and exhaled. I didn't realize I'd been holding my breath.

He extracted the tube, which was quick and painless. The whole procedure had lasted only a few minutes. Looking pleased, Dr. Peters asked if I was taking medicine for my prostate.

"Dr. Uro has me on Avodart twice a week."

"I suggest you take it every day," he said. "I don't see any need to see you again unless you feel the need for a follow-up visit."

"With all due respect, doctor, I'd rather not."

He patted me on the shoulder.

"I'm glad this worked out so well for you," he said as he left the room, presumably to perform the same procedure on someone else. If so, I hoped the outcome was just as happy.

I exited the procedure room feeling like I was walking on air. As soon as I saw Elvira, I gave her the thumbs-up. As we walked out of the office, I told her about my king-sized prostate and its intrusion into my bladder. She was just as thrilled as I was, and the weight that had settled on us over the past twenty-four hours was lifted.

Ten days later, we would have a great Christmas that was as meaningful as any in our lives. We celebrated, full of hope for the future. On New Year's Eve, Elvira and I opened a bottle of champagne and toasted to good health and many more years together.

THE STORY CONTINUES

This is not the end of the story. It would have been if I'd died before the end of 2016, which seemed likely when we first heard my diagnosis in May. The story might also end here if I had been cancer-free by the end of the year, or even if the cancer had gone into remission. That was not the case. The immunotherapy drugs had been effective but not effective enough to rid me completely of my melanoma.

Now that I think of it, remission would not have ended the story. As Dr. Onco had pointed out, cancer could always return. Even when the cancer was invisible, it could still be in my system, waiting for an opportunity to attack again.

But I wasn't even that far along in the process because I still had traces of the melanoma on my liver and kidney. I was not cancer-free, and as we were reminded by the bladder scare, cancer was unpredictable. Dr. Onco had also admitted that he didn't know what effect immunotherapy had on new cancers. He seemed to think bladder cancer was a distinct possibility when he saw the shadow on my CT scan because immunotherapy was monogamous. The Yervoy-Opdivo regimen was designed to combat only the metastatic melanoma.

This was the negative side. It is important to describe fully because I want to explain why I'm stopping my journal at this point and why I want to continue in another, more open-ended venue.

Before I get to the positives, however, I need to mention side effects as more evidence of the negative side. Before I started the immunotherapy, the NP had presented a long list of potential side effects. Both she and Dr. Onco had admitted that I might get sick from the regimen. And, of course, I did. Among other things, I lost 30 pounds and was clearly on a downward spiral during the second half of the combination treatments. The side effects were as unpredictable as the cancer, maybe more. In addition, the recent article in *The New York Times* had pointed out that serious side effects could occur long after the treatment stops.

All of that is on one side. Now, I'll get to the positives. The list may not be as long, but it's powerful.

First and foremost, I was alive. I ate a hearty Thanksgiving meal, celebrated Christmas with family and friends, hugged my wife at midnight on New Year's Eve, and went out to a scrumptious dinner with Elvira on our anniversary on January 2. These were important landmarks for me, this year more than ever.

Plus, even though I was not in remission, my partial response had improved my condition and promised to continue to improve it. It seemed as if every day, I was living more like I had before I got sick, and so was Elvira. Thanks to the immunotherapy, we had made amazing progress over the course of seven months and were grateful beyond words.

Which is why I've decided to end the journal here. I've said enough about how sick I was, how I got sicker before getting better, and how wonderful it was to make progress toward a healthier life. To continue that trend, Dr. Onco will keep me on Opdivo until it either stops working or the cancer becomes undetectable. Even if I go into remission, he said he would order regular CT scans to make sure the melanoma did not make an unceremonious return.

This is the end of my journal, but the story continues. By the time this journal is published, I intend to have a blog entitled "Melanoma without a Cause" for anyone who wishes to read more about my life as an immunotherapy patient. My hope is that it contains nothing more than a weekly chronicle of how good I feel and how much fun Elvira and I are having. In other words, I hope it's boring as hell.

But you never know.

ABOUT THE AUTHOR

Bryant Wieneke has written an eclectic set of non-fiction and fiction books, beginning with the publication of *Winning Without the Spin*, an insider's account of a visionary religious studies professor's campaign for Congress. His second full-length work was his comical Peace Corps journal, set in West Africa. Following the publication of *Melanoma without a Cause*, Mr. Wieneke will return to his personal biography series, books that allow the reader to join historical figures on their journeys of discovery, and his contemporary novels that explore peaceful means of deterring or pre-empting terrorism. A former university administrator, Mr. Wieneke retired in 2013 to devote himself to writing.

Made in the
USA
Middletown, DE